EAT ME
SOUTH SHORE

MASSACHUSETTS GUIDE TO LOCAL, ORGANIC,
AND SUSTAINABLE FOOD, FARMS, AND FARMERS
MARKETS ON THE SOUTH SHORE.

BY NOREEN FINNERAN

First Printing: 2018 LULU

ISBN 978-0-359-10133-7

Check out the Eat Me South Shore Blog:
https://eatmesouthshorema.blogspot.com/

Find other books by Noreen Finneran:
http://www.lulu.com/spotlight/finneran

EAT ME SOUTH SHORE:

MASSACHUSETTS GUIDE TO LOCAL, ORGANIC, AND SUSTAINABLE FOOD, FARMS, AND FARMERS MARKETS ON THE SOUTH SHORE

WRITTEN BY NOREEN FINNERAN

Contents

Eat Me, South Shore

Massachusetts guide to local, organic, and sustainable food, farms, and farmers markets on the South Shore.

INTRO

Do you want to eat local, organic, and sustainable food? Do you like to support your local farmers and artisans? Do you want to avoid buying food that contains GMO's, chemicals or pesticides? Do you want to support farms that practice and promote humane farming practices? Do you want to visit more local farms and farmers markets this year? Well, then you have come to the right place.

I always want to eat local, organic, or sustainably farmed food. But, not knowing where to look or when to look for my favorites has left me failing. It seems that whenever I actually get out to my local farmers market there is nothing but lettuce and tomatoes at an exorbitant price. That is probably because I am going to the wrong place at the wrong time of year. But, then what is the best place and best time of year? How do I find out where to go? Also, how do I know which farms are organic or sustainable?

The goal of this book is to answer all those questions and make it easier for all of us on the South Shore to get to a farm or farmers market and get the best quality produce at the peak of the season. The second goal is to find local farms that practice organic, humane and sustainable farming practices. The third goal is to find organic or sustainable farms that cleanly grow what are known as the "dirty dozen" and GMO foods.

FARMING PRACTICES

It is useful to know the farming practices of your local farm. Most farmers do not have the time or wherewithal to inform customers of their farming methods. Also their methods may change from year to year. Other times they don't know the proper label for their methods. Even if they did announce their practices some customers wouldn't know the meaning of their method.

What are the most common farming practices of today? To start, I will break them down from the most stringent practices to the most lenient. We have *USDA certified organic* at the top followed by *Certified Naturally Grown* and *uncertified organic* and *sustainable farming* right behind with *conventional farming* at the bottom.

Which farming method should I look for when buying from my local farm? Which farming method is best? Is it worth the extra cost to buy locally and organic or sustainable? Which label will guarantee little to no chemicals on my produce? Is an organic local farm apple better than a sustainable local farm apple? What about a conventional local farm? Spoiler alert: you can buy from all of these farms with the possible exception of the conventional farm for a high quality, environmentally-friendly, healthy, low or chemical-free product. In my opinion, even a conventional local farm is a healthier and smarter choice than conventional produce from the supermarket.

Let's start with the United States Department of Agriculture (USDA), *Certified Organic* label. This is the most strict and bureaucratic label for a farmer to achieve. It is also the most expensive and time-consuming to maintain. This means higher prices for the farmer and consumer. Farmers must follow strict guidelines to obtain this label. For example, the land must be free from synthetic pesticides, a USDA-approved agent must inspect regularly and sometimes randomly, animal welfare approval is necessary, no GMO's are allowed, farmers must use specific organic pesticides, they must go through the process to obtain *Organic Certification*, they must keep good records for the USDA, they must adhere to the National list of *Allowed And Prohibited Substances*, and they must use well water if town water is treated by a prohibited substance. The guidelines farmers must follow in order to obtain USDA *Organic Certification* labelling seem endless. This stringency is good for us, the consumers. We are guaranteed to get a product that uses no synthetic pesticides (but they may use organic pesticides), no GMO's, and no prohibited substances. [i]

Some farms practice organic methods but don't obtain their certification. They call themselves *uncertified organic farms*. Silverbrook Farm of Dartmouth put it best, "We decided not to be a certified organic farm. The paper trail, record keeping and additional clerical procedures required became overwhelming. We applaud those who can complete these tasks! We plan to farm with responsible and sustainable methods but not go through the certification process. This means lower costs for us and helps us keep our prices in line with other producers (a very important aspect for customers)." They also eloquently explain why it is worth spending more money on organic and sustainable produce, "Why some farmers charge more is because instead of taking easy, short term solutions like spraying a field with toxic weed killers, a sustainable farmer needs to mulch, weed-whack (string trim) or hand weed. Many such practices are more labor intensive than conventional methods. However, we do believe that in the long term sustainable agriculture has less cost involved – no sick workers, no polluted water and no harmful residue on food. We also pay our employees a livable wage which factors into our market costs." [ii] Certified Organic or sustainable farmers pay fees to maintain certification which could raise the cost of their produce.

What does it mean to be *Certified Naturally Grown*? Some farmers want to be sustainable with a certification but can't or don't want to deal with the bureaucracy of the USDA Organic processes. These farmers opt for the *Certified Naturally Grown* (CNG) label instead. The CNG label is a peer-review program. The CNG program requires farmers to pay membership dues, sign a *Declaration of Terms*, and allow on-site inspections by other CNG farmers. CNG farmers must also keep records of receipts, purchases, applications, soil test results, etc. They need to re-certify every year. The declaration states that the farmer has been free of using prohibited synthetic pesticides, herbicides and fertilizers for at least three years (36 months) from the date of their first saleable harvest. [iii] They are inspected and questioned about their tillage practices, erosion control practices, crop rotation practices, manure and compost management, irrigation sources, water conservation, etc. CNG farmers are allowed to use specific substances including essential oils, minerals, compost, biological and microbial products, and cover crops. [iv] They are not allowed to use any GMO seeds, GMO crops, synthetic substances, prohibited non-synthetic substances, ionizing radiation, and sewage sludge. So, if you buy from a *Certified Naturally Grown* farm you are guaranteed to get a product with no synthetic pesticides, no GMO's, and no prohibited substances. On top of that, you are guaranteed to support a farmer that uses best environmental practices and sustainable methods.

Then, what does it mean to be a sustainable farm? This label is open to interpretation but all the previously listed farms are sustainable farms. That means that the certified organic, uncertified organic, certified naturally grown, and sustainable farms are all good for you and the earth. A sustainable farmer uses little to no pesticides. If they do, they use eco-friendly pesticides and only when necessary or as a last resort. Sustainable farmers practice methods such as crop rotation, using cover crops, utilizing Integrated Pest Management (IPM) practices, hand weeding, recycling, and composting that help protect or preserve the land and water. Sustainable farmers work according to their philosophy but don't require a certification or inspection for that title. That gives the farmer more time to work the farm rather than fill out paperwork. As consumers, we trust the sustainable farmer at their word. When you buy from a sustainable farm you are likely getting a product with no synthetic pesticides, no GMO's, and no prohibited substances. On top of that, your purchase supports the farmer that uses best environmental farm practices and sustainable methods.

Check out Consumer Reports website, *Greener Choices*, for a more in-depth look at food labels such as; organic, pasture-raised, cruelty-free, free-range, certified humane raised and handled, etc.[v]

DIRTY DOZEN & GMOS

If we are on a budget and can't afford to buy everything organic, what organically or sustainably farmed products should we buy? Where can we find local farms that grow these items? I don't mind paying more money if it's worth it. And I believe that it's worth paying more for locally and sustainably grown produce that would otherwise be full of chemicals when bought conventionally at the supermarket. If you are like me then this next chapter is worth a read.

Certain products are more susceptible to disease, rot, or insect infestation and require more pesticides and insecticides to produce a saleable yield crop. Unfortunately, those pesticides leach into the ground, water, and eventually our bodies when we eat those crops. Over a dozen conventionally grown crops have tested positive for high pesticide residue and have been deemed the *"Dirty Dozen"*. These items should be bought organically or sustainably farmed in order to get the cleanest product. Below is a list of the "Dirty Dozen" in order of *dirtiest* aka highest chemical residue left on the plant to least dirty (as of 2018):

Strawberries
Spinach
Nectarines
Apples
Peaches
Celery
Grapes

Pears
Cherries
Tomatoes
Sweet bell peppers
Potatoes
Green Beans, lettuce and Kale are making it up this list also.

As if that were not bad enough we should also avoid GMO's. GMO's are Genetically Modified Organisms. Genetic modification is radically different than farmer or bee modification i.e. cross pollination, grafting, or cross breeding.

According to the U.S. Food and Drug Administration [FDA], Genetically Modified Organisms aka GMOs or genetic engineering of food is when, "scientists make targeted changes to a plant's genetic makeup to give the plant a new desirable trait." [vi] Sometimes this means taking a gene from an organism that is not remotely related to the final product. In other words, it is creating an entirely new organism.

Farmers have been modifying plant breeds for years but in a way that mimics nature. Farmers work with plants in the field and cross-breed by transferring pollen from one plant to another, much like a bee does.

To make a GMO, scientists isolate one desirable gene and add it to a single plant cell in a laboratory to generate a new plant from that cell. This new plant now contains that isolated gene creating a new plant variety. That desirable gene could have come from a fish. A farmer or a bee could not achieve this goal in the natural world.

Some GMO crops are modified to tolerate higher levels of pesticides meaning more pesticides can now be used on those crops. It is thought that those pesticides remain on and in the crops that we eat. Glyphosate commonly known as *Roundup* is a pesticide believed to be a human carcinogen.

According to the U.S. Food and Drug Administration [FDA], there are only a handful of GMOs on the market; Cotton, corn, soybeans, potatoes, squash, apples and papayas. But, they are processed to make ingredients such as;

Canola
Canola oil
Corn oil
Corn starch
Corn Syrup
Cottonseed oil
Granulated sugar
High-fructose corn syrup
Soy lecithin
Soybean oil

These Genetically Modified [GM] ingredients are commonly found in commercial soups, sauces, mayonnaise, salad dressings, breads, snack foods, and much more.[vii]

These GMO crops are often hidden from the consumer under the new ingredient name. For example, GMO corn is used to produce **high-fructose corn syrup** and **corn starch** that is found in a multitude of food and drinks. GMO Soybeans are used to produce **soy lecithin** which is present in products including **dark chocolate and candy bars**. GMO Cotton is used to produce **cottonseed oil** used in **potato chips** and **margarine**. **Canola** is used to produce oil for cooking as well as emulsifiers used in packaged foods. GMO **Sugar beets** are used in the production of **granulated sugar**. If any of these ingredients are listed on the package then you are likely ingesting a GMO unless otherwise noted.[viii]

Here is a current list of commercial crops that are genetically modified, genetic traits of the new organism and the year they were first launched[ix]:

Squash, Disease resistance, 1995
Cotton, Herbicide Tolerance, Insect resistance, 1996
Soybean, Herbicide Tolerance, Insect resistance, 1995
Corn, Insect resistance, Herbicide Tolerance, drought tolerance, 1996
Papaya, Disease resistance, 1997
Alfalfa, Herbicide Tolerance, 2006
Sugar beets, Herbicide Tolerance, 2006
Canola, Herbicide Tolerance, 1999
Potato, non-browning, reduced bruising, low acrylamide, blight resistance, 2016
Apples, non-browning, 2017

To assure that you are not eating GMO's you must buy organic or look for the *non GMO* labelling. Some products have "Non GMO Project Verified" stickers on their packaging. The Non GMO Project has an app enabling you to scan barcodes for GMO information.[x]

Below is an alphabetical list of foods that should be grown and bought organically or sustainably because they are one of the dirty dozen, known for high pesticide residue, or could be a GMO:

Alfalfa
Apples
Beans, Green
Beets (Sugar)
Celery
Cherries
Corn
Grapes
Kale
Nectarines
Papaya
Peaches
Pears
Peppers, Sweet bell
Potatoes
Soybean
Spinach
Squash
Strawberries
Tomatoes

ORGANIC PRODUCE FINDER

Now you know which produce to buy organically but can you find them locally grown? Yes, you can find most of these crops on the South Shore. Some farms are certified organic and others use sustainable farming practices. Both types of farms are better than conventional farms. But local conventional farms are still a better choice than supermarket farms.

So, where can you find these "dirty" items locally and organically or sustainably farmed? Below is a list of some local farms that are environmentally responsible and grow one or more of the following dirty dozen or GMO crops.

Always call or check out the farm's website or Facebook page for the most up-to-date information. See the FARMS chapter for full details on each farm:

ALFALFA

Freedom Food Farm

APPLES

Peak season is approximately August to October.

Barden Family Orchard

Colchester Neighborhood Farm

Elliot Farm

Elwood Orchard

Peachtree Circle Farm

Russell Orchards

Silverbrook Farms

BEANS, GREEN

Peak season is approximately June to October.

C&C Reading Farm

Colchester Neighborhood Farm

Elliot Farm

Holly Hill Farm

Langwater Farm

Second Nature Farm

Skinny Dip Farm

BEETS (SUGAR)

Peak season is approximately mid-June to mid-October.

C&C Reading Farm

Cape Cod Organic Farm

Colchester Neighborhood Farm

Holly Hill Farm

Peachtree Circle Farm

Second Nature Farm

Silverbrook Farms

Skinny Dip Farm

CELERY

Peak season is approximately late-July to November.

Brix Bounty Farm

C&C Reading Farm

Colchester Neighborhood Farm

Freedom Food Farm

Natick Community Organic Farm

Russell Orchards

Second Nature Farm

CHERRIES

Peak season is approximately mid-June to early-July.

Russell Orchards

Ward's Berry Farm

Web of Life Organic Farm

CORN

Peak season is approximately July to mid-October.

Barden Family Orchard

C&C Reading Farm

C.N. Smith Farm

Colchester Neighborhood Farm

E.L. Silvia Farms

Elliot Farm

Langwater Farm

Plimoth Grist Mill

Silverbrook Farms

GRAPES

Peak season is approximately August to September.

Agraria Farm

Russell Orchards

KALE

Peak season is approximately mid-May to October.

Brix Bounty Farm

Cape Cod Organic Farm

Colchester Neighborhood Farm

Freedom Food Farm

Holly Hill Farm

Russell Orchards

Second Nature Farm

Silverbrook Farms

Skinny Dip Farm

NECTARINES

Peak season is approximately August to September.

E.L. Silvia Farms

Elwood Orchard

Russell Orchards

PAPAYA

Papayas are not traditionally grown in New England. Peak season in Florida is approximately December to May, limited in June.[xi] Avoid conventional papayas grown in Hawaii and certain varieties like: *Rainbow papayas*, *Sun Up Strawberry*, and *Sunrise* as these are common GMOs. Instead choose organic from Florida, Mexico or Belize and/or these varieties; Kapoho aka Kapoho Solo, The Mexican Red, Caribbean Red, Maradol, Royal Star Papayas, Florida Red Royale, the Singapore Pink, and the Higgins variety.[xii]

Whole Foods Market

Miami Fruit

PEACHES

Peak season is approximately mid-July to mid-September.

Barden Family Orchard

Colchester Neighborhood Farm

E.L. Silvia Farms

Elliot Farm

Elwood Orchard

Langwater Farm

Peachtree Circle Farm

Russell Orchards

Silverbrook Farms

Ward's Berry Farm

PEARS

Peak season is approximately September to mid-November.

Elwood Orchard

Peachtree Circle Farm

Russell Orchards

PEPPERS, SWEET BELL

Peak season is approximately July through October.

Brix Bounty Farm

C&C Reading Farm

Cape Cod Organic Farm

Colchester Neighborhood Farm

Elliot Farm

Langwater Farm

Nest and Song Farm

Peachtree Circle Farm

Second Nature Farm

Silverbrook Farms

Skinny Dip Farm

Web Of Life Farm

POTATOES

Peak season is approximately August to November.

C&C Reading Farm

Cape Cod Organic Farm

Elliot Farm

Freedom Food Farm

Holly Hill Farm

Langwater Farm

Nest and Song Farm

Peachtree Circle Farm

Russell Orchards

Second Nature Farm

Silverbrook Farms

Skinny Dip Farm

SOYBEAN

Soybeans are not traditionally grown in New England. [xiii]
Look for ones grown in North Carolina, Ohio, Indiana,
Kentucky and Illinois. Harvest season is approximately
October through November.

Whole Foods

Your local natural food store

SPINACH

Peak season is approximately May through October.

Brix Bounty Farm

C&C Reading Farm

Colchester Neighborhood Farm

Freedom Food Farm

Langwater Farm

Russell Orchards

Second Nature Farm

Skinny Dip Farm

SQUASH

Peak season is approximately July to Mid-October for Summer Squash and September through November for Winter Squash.

Barden Family Orchard

Brix Bounty Farm

C&C Reading Farm

Cape Cod Organic Farm

Elliot Farm

Freedom Food Farm

Langwater Farm

Peachtree Circle Farm

Second Nature Farm

Skinny Dip Farm

STRAWBERRIES

Peak season is approximately late-May through June. Strawberries can be found as late as August some years.

Agraria Farm

Allen Farms

Brix Bounty Farm

C&C Reading Farm

Freedom Food Farm

Langwater Farm

Nest and Song Farm

Russell Orchards

Second Nature Farm

Silverbrook Farms

Ward's Berry Farm

Wise Acre Farm

TOMATOES

Peak season is approximately mid-August to Mid-October.

Brix Bounty Farm

C&C Reading Farm

Cape Cod Organic Farm

Colchester Neighborhood Farm

E.L. Silvia Farms

Elliot Farm

Freedom Food Farm

Holly Hill Farm

Langwater Farm

Peachtree Circle Farm

Second Nature Farm

Silverbrook Farms

Skinny Dip Farm

Web Of Life Farm

White Gate Gardens

DIRTY DOZEN GMO CALENDAR

When searching for seasonal, organic or sustainable "dirty" produce look for kale and spinach in the spring followed by strawberries, beans, beets, and cherries. Then, by mid-summer look for celery, corn, peaches, peppers, and summer squash. Late-summer brings apples, grapes, nectarines, potatoes, and tomatoes. Fall brings more apples and pears. Look for soybeans and papaya late fall and into our winter but they will have to be bought from distant farms as they don't grow well in this region.

JAN	FEB	MAR	APR	MAY	JUN	JUL	AUG	SEP	OCT	NOV	DEC
							Apples	Apples	Apples		
					Beans	Beans	Beans	Beans	Beans		
					Beets	Beets	Beets	Beets	Beets		
						Celery	Celery	Celery	Celery	Celery	
					Cherries	Cherries					
						Corn	Corn	Corn	Corn		
							Grapes	Grapes			
			Kale	Kale	Kale	Kale	Kale	Kale	Kale		
							Nectarines	Nectarines			
Papaya	Papaya	Papaya	Papaya								Papaya
						Peaches	Peaches	Peaches			
								Pears	Pears	Pears	
					Peppers	Peppers	Peppers	Peppers	Peppers		
							Potatoes	Potatoes	Potatoes	Potatoes	
									Soybean	Soybean	
			Spinach	Spinach	Spinach	Spinach	Spinach	Spinach	Spinach		
					Squash	Squash	Squash	Squash	Squash		
				Strawberries							
							Tomatoes	Tomatoes	Tomatoes		

SPECIALTY PRODUCE CALENDAR

	JAN	FEB	MAR	APR	MAY	JUN	JUL	AUG	SEP	OCT	NOV	DEC
Black Trumpet Mushroom	X	X	X									X
Chanterelle Mushroom	X	X		X	X	X	X					
Cherries						X	X	X				
Cranberries										X	X	
Currants							X					
Elderberry						X	X					
Fennel									X	X	X	X
Fiddleheads				X								
Figs						X			X			
Garlic Scapes					X	X						
Ginger							X	X				
Gooseberries						X	X					
Grapes								X	X			
Hedgehog Mushroom	X									X		
Horseradish				X					X	X		
Jostaberries							X					
Kohlrabi						X			X	X		
Lingonberries									X			
Lobster Mushroom							X	X				
Matsutake Mushroom									X	X		
Morels				X	X							
Nectarines							X	X				
Parsnips			X							X		
Peaches							X	X				
Pears								X	X			
Plums							X	X				
Porcini Mushroom						X			X			
Purslane						X	X					
Quince										X	X	
Ramps				X	X							
Raspberries							X					
Rhubarb				X	X							
Soybeans								X				
Strawberries						X						
Sunchokes						X						
Tomatillos								X	X			
Tomatoes								X	X			
White Truffle Mushroom	X										X	
	JAN	FEB	MAR	APR	MAY	JUN	JUL	AUG	SEP	OCT	NOV	DEC

29

FARMS

It can be expensive, time consuming, labor intensive, and risky to grow crops using organic or sustainable farming practices. But, even still I have found local farmers who have risen to the challenge.

Some farms offer a U-Pick or Pick Your Own option aka PYO. Check their website for details and the most up-to-date information.

Many of the farms offer Farm Boxes, Farm Shares, or Community Supported Agriculture aka CSA. When you sign up for a Farm Box, Farm Share, or CSA you are ensuring an income for the farmer and the freshest available produce for yourself.

Farm information changes frequently so it is recommended to call or visit the farm's Facebook page or website before visiting. The top organic or sustainable farms in and around the South Shore, include (but are not limited to):

Agraria Farm, 17 Willard Ave., Rehoboth, MA 02769. Phone: 508-336-3823. Organic Farm. This farm grows flowers, fruit, herbs, mushrooms, vegetables, organic eggs, rhubarb, strawberries, blueberries, raspberries, blackberries, grapes, elderberries, gooseberries, jostaberries, currants, lingonberries, figs, and melons. http://www.agrariafarm.com

Alderbrook Farm, 1213 Russells Mills Road, Dartmouth, MA. Phone: 774-264-0755. Sustainable Farm. This farm grows flowers, herbs, corn, zucchini, radishes, cucumbers, beets, honey, maple syrup, eggs, and milk, etc.

Allen Farms, 913 Division Rd, Dartmouth, MA 02748. Organic Farm. This farm grows flowers, herbs, seedlings, vegetables, lettuce, tomatoes, strawberries & wineberries. Find them at the following farmers markets: Chatham, Falmouth, Osterville, and Provincetown, Pawtucket, Plimoth Plantation, & Marshfield. http://www.allenfarmsorganics.com

Apponagansett Farm, 607 Elm Street, Dartmouth, MA 02748. Phone: 774-400-7277. Sustainable Farm. This farm grows salad greens, spinach, root crops, potatoes, brassicas, beans, tomatoes, watermelon, cantaloupe, melons, strawberries, fennel, leeks, winter squash, pumpkins, herbs, flowers, pasture raised chicken eggs, etc. CSA available. Farm stand is open from June - November 10:00 AM -7:00 PM. Find them at the following farmers markets: Dartmouth, New Bedford, Pawtucket wintertime, New Bedford Indoor market, and at several local natural food stores. http://www.apponagansettfarm.com/

At Cranberry Hill, 103 Haskell Rd, Plymouth, MA 02360. Phone: 508-888-9179. Organic cranberry farm. This farm grows cranberries. They take orders all summer long at cranhill@capecod.net or by phone or fax at 508-888-9179. http://organiccranberries.com/

Barden Family Orchard, 56 Elmdale Rd North Scituate, RI 02857. Phone: 401-934-1413. Sustainable Farm. IPM practices. This farm grows apples, pumpkins, winter squash, peaches, sweet corn, raspberries, blueberries, tomatoes, summer squash, zucchini, cucumbers and eggplant. Open by appointment only at the farm. Farm Market is open Monday thru Friday 9:00 AM -6:00 PM and Saturday and Sunday 9:00 AM -5:00 PM. Find them at the following farmers markets: Find them at Coastal Growers Market, Pawtucket Wintertime Market, and Aquidneck Growers Market. http://bardenfamilyorchard.com/

Bay End Farm, 200 Bournedale Rd., Bourne, MA. Phone: 617-212-8315. Organic Farm. CSA available. This farm grows organic vegetables, herbs, and flowers. Farm stand is open Tuesdays, Thursdays, and Fridays from 11:00 AM - 6:00 PM, Wednesdays from 12:30 PM -6:00 PM and Saturdays from 10:00 AM -4:00 PM through mid-October. http://www.bayendfarm.com/farmstand/

Blackbird Farm, 660 Douglas Pike, Smithfield, RI 02917. Phone: 401-232-2495. Sustainable Farm. This farm grows humanely raised all-natural, hormone-free, pasture-fed, 100% Black Angus cattle; 100% pedigreed American Heritage Berkshire pigs; and organic, free-range Rhode Island Red eggs. Farm stand is open Thursday and Friday 1:00 PM -6:00 PM, Saturday 9:00 AM -6:00 PM, Sunday 9:00 AM -4:00 PM. They host their own farmers market at their farm stand on Fridays 3:00 PM -6:00 PM beginning in the summer until end of October. Vendors at their farmers market include; Steere Orchard, Aquidneck Honey etc. https://blackbirdfarmri.com/

Brix Bounty Farm, 449 Bakerville Road, Dartmouth, MA. Phone: 508-992-1868. Sustainable Farm. Brix Bounty's produce is grown without chemical pesticides or herbicides. This farm grows celery, kale, squash, zucchini, lettuce, peppers, spinach, tomatoes, tomatillos, strawberries, etc. CSA available. Farm stand is open weekends in the spring & daily in the summer 10:00 AM until dusk until November. Find them at the following farmers markets: New Bedford. http://www.brixbounty.com/

Brown Boar Farm, 543 Lamb Hill Road, East Wells, VT 05774. Phone: 802-325-2461. Sustainable Farm. They raise heritage pork and beef, sustainable, free- range and cruelty-free. Find them at the following farmers markets: Marshfield Fair, South Shore Winter Farmers Market Scituate, and Plymouth Farmers Market. They can be found in local stores including Simpson Spring in Easton, MA. http://www.brownboarfarm.com/

C&C Reading Farm, LLC., formerly Billingsgate Farm, 175 East Center Street, West Bridgewater, MA. Phone: 781-293-6144 or 508-857-0657. Partially organic farm and the rest is a sustainable farm. PYO available strawberries in June- bring your own container or use theirs. This farm grows herbs, vegetables, popcorn, beans, beets, blueberries, broccoli, celery, corn, cucumbers, potatoes, spinach, strawberries, tomatoes, squash etc. CSA available. Farm stand hours: Monday – Friday 10:00 AM – 6:30 PM, Saturday & Sunday 9:00 AM – 6:30 PM. PYO open daily June through October from

10:00 AM -6:30 PM.   Corn mazes, wagon rides and pumpkin patch. http://www.ccreadingfarm.com/

Cape Abilities Farm, 458 Route 6A, Dennis, MA. Phone: 508-385-2538. Sustainable Farm. This farm grows tomatoes, cucumbers, lettuce, etc. This farm works to provide skills and jobs for individuals with disabilities. Farm open every day from 9:30 AM-5:00 PM. Farm store at 193 Main St., Chatham, MA, open Wednesday to Saturday 9:00 AM-5:00 PM, Sundays 10:00AM-5:00PM. http://www.capeabilities.org/

Cape Cod Organic Farm, (Rt. 6A), 3675 Main St Barnstable, MA 02630. Phone: 508-362-3573. Organic Farm. This farm grows berries, seed potatoes, seedlings, vegetables, organic heritage breed piglets, and pork. CSA available. Farm stand is open every day 9:30 AM to 4:30 PM, Wednesday 9:30 AM-5:30 PM. Find them at the following farmers markets: Orleans, Wellfleet and Truro Farmers Markets. http://www.capecodorganicfarm.org/

Cape Cod Select, 73 Tremont St., Carver, MA. Phone: 508-866-1149. Sustainable Farm. Solar powered facilities. This farm grows cranberries from flower to package. The farm's premium frozen cranberries are available year-round in gourmet food stores and supermarkets throughout the U.S. including your local Shaw's, Stop & Shop, and Good Health Natural Foods. https://www.capecodselect.com

Choke Cherry Farm, 80 North St., Duxbury, MA. Phone: 781-837-2121. Organic Farm. This farm grows vegetables, tomatoes, lettuce, garlic, peppers, etc. Find at The Market at Pinehills in Plymouth. https://www.theorganicfoodguide.org/

Cluck and Trowel, 875 Horseneck Road, Westport, MA. Phone: 508-542-6451. Certified Organic Farm. This farm grows organic herbs, onions, tomatoes, cucumbers, pastured chicken eggs, etc. CSA available and Farm Boxes available. Find them at the following farmers markets: Pawtucket Wintertime Farmers Market. Find seasonally at the self-serve stand at 777 Horseneck Rd, South Dartmouth, MA. Check their website or Facebook page to see what is available each week. http://www.cluckandtrowel.com/

C.N. Smith Farm, Inc., 325 South St., East Bridgewater, MA. Phone: 508-378-2270. Sustainable Farm. They don't spray pesticides on their fruit but they do spray the trees at the start and end of the season. PYO strawberries, blueberries, peaches, raspberries, apples, pumpkins. PYO hours vary so make sure to call ahead. Currently PYO hours for apples are Wednesday-Friday 10:00AM-4:00PM, Weekends 9:00AM-4:00PM (times are subject to change from product to product and season to season). This farm sells eggs, cider donuts, sweet corn, lettuce, peaches, plums, nectarines, pears, tomatoes, etc. They have a farm stand open from March thru December, 9:00 AM -5:00 PM Sunday and Monday and 9:00 AM -6:00 PM Tuesday thru Saturday. They also have a Garden Center. http://cnsmithfarminc.com

Colchester Neighborhood Farm, 90 Brook Street, Plympton, MA 02367. Phone: 781-422-3921. Organic Farm. This farm grows apples, beans (green), beets (sugar), celery, corn, kale, peaches, peppers (sweet bell), spinach, tomatoes, etc. CSA available. Farm stand is open seven days a week in the winter from 10:00 AM -3:00 PM and in the summer from 10:00 AM -6:00 PM. Find them at the following farmers markets: Plymouth Farmers Market in Plimoth Plantation. The farm is community driven and employs intellectually and developmentally challenged adults. http://www.colchesterneighborhoodfarm.com

Copicut Farms, 11 Copicut Road, North Dartmouth, MA. Sustainable Farm. This farm raises pasture-raised, humanely processed, non GMO fed, pork, beef, turkeys, chicken, and eggs. Farm Shares available. Farm Store open Saturdays June through November from 10:00 AM - 4:00 PM. They offer home delivery in eastern Mass. Find at Lees market in Westport, Mass. Find them at the following farmers markets: Boston area farmers markets, Milton Farmers Market, Plymouth Plantation Farmers Market, Dartmouth Farmers Market, and Hingham Farmers Market. https://www.copicutfarms.com/

Cretinon's Farm Stand, 86 Landing Rd, Kingston, MA 02364. Phone: 781-585-5531. Sustainable Farm. This farm is not certified organic but it uses organic and sustainable methods. This farm grows lettuce, strawberries, asparagus, etc. Find them at the following farmers markets: Carver, Cohasset, and Marshfield.

DaSilva Farm, 430 Jepson Lane, Portsmouth, RI. Phone: 401-528-9442. Sustainable Farm. This farm raises pasture-raised, chicken, eggs, turkey, pork and eggs. CSA available. Farm stand is open June to November, call for hours. This farm partners with Norwell Farms and Holly Hill Farm, Cohasset. Find them at the following farmers markets: Braintree, Marshfield, Plymouth, Crescent Ridge, and SoWa Farmers Market in Boston. http://www.dasilvafarm.com/#home-page

Deep Roots Farm, 77 Victory Highway, Chepachet, RI. Phone: 510-410-3268. Sustainable Farm. This farm raises pasture-raised, chemical-free, beef, pork, eggs, and chickens. CSA available. Open Wednesday 3:00 PM -6:00 PM and Saturday 9:00 AM -noon. https://deeprootsfarm.org/

Dufort Farms, 55 Reservoir Ave, Rehoboth, MA, 02769. Phone: 508-252-6323. Organic and Sustainable Farm. PYO blueberries available in July. This farm raises organic turkeys, sustainable berries, grass-fed beef, pigs foraged outside, and eggs. Farm stand is open Saturdays 8:00 AM -4:00 PM. Find them at the following farmers markets: Plymouth Farmers Market at Plimoth Plantation. Note: NO RESTROOMS ON FARM. http://www.dufortfarms.com/

Earthwright Farm, Holbrook, MA. Sustainable farm that does not use chemicals on their produce. They grow strawberries, blueberries, etc. Find them at the following farmers markets: Randolph Farmers Market.

E & T Farms, 85 Lombard Ave., West Barnstable, MA 02668. Phone: 508-362-8370. Sustainable Farm. This farm grows edible flowers, micro greens, honey, farm raised shrimp, hydroponic vegetables, etc. Farm Store open Monday-Friday 8:30 AM -4:30 PM. Find them at the Dennis Organic Market, Mashpee Organic Market, Chatham Organic Market, Barnstable Market and Orleans Whole Foods. Dehttp://eandtfarmsinc.com/products_shrimp.htm

E.L. Silvia Farms, 2621 County St., Dighton, MA. Phone: 508-982-8612. Sustainable Farm uses IPM. This farm grows corn, nectarines, tomatoes, and peaches, etc. Find them at the following farmers markets: Scituate Farmers Market.

Elliot Farm, 202 Main Street, Lakeville, MA 02347. Phone: 508-947-5954. Sustainable Farm. This farm grows corn, tomatoes, squash, cucumbers, peppers, apples, peaches, cantaloupe, veggies sold in season only. CSA available. Farm stand is open daily 10:00 AM -6:00 PM from July to September. https://www.elliotfarm.org

Elwood Orchard, 58 Snake Hill Road, North Scituate, RI 02857. Phone: 401-949-0390. Organic Farm. PYO organic apples available. This farm grows organic apples, garlic, shallots, shitake mushrooms, Asian pears, and sustainable stone fruit (nectarines, peaches and plums) grown with organic pesticides. Farm Store open seasonally seven days a week from 9:00 AM -5:00 PM. Check their website or Facebook page for what is available each week. http://www.elwoodorchard.com/

Foxboro Cheese Co., on Lawton's Family Farm, 70 North St, in Foxboro, MA. Phone: 508-543-6460. Sustainable Farm. This farm sells grass-fed beef and veal, raw milk, Asiago and Fromage Blanc cheese made from their own grass-fed grazing Ayrshire cow's milk. Farm stand is open 10:00 AM -6:00 PM. Find them at the following farmers markets: Hingham, Scituate, Marshfield, Norwood, and Wayland Winter Farmers Market.
https://foxborocheeseco.wordpress.com/

Freedom Food Farm, 471 Leonard St, Raynham, MA 02767. Phone: 978-884-7102. Sustainable Farm. Holistic farming practices. This farm grows vegetables, celery, kale, potatoes, spinach, squash, strawberries, tomatoes, grains, herbs, strawberries, flowers, hay, pasture, seedlings, eggs, laying hens, pasture-raised meat, beef, broiler chickens, turkeys, hogs, pork, lamb, goat, etc. CSA available. Farm Store is open year-round Wednesday to Saturday from 10-6, closed Sunday, Monday, and Tuesday. Summer hours differ May through December, call ahead. Find them at the following farmers markets: Pawtucket, Somerville, and Attleboro Farmers Market. They are partnered with Norwell farms CSA. They offer hayrides and workshops.
http://www.freedomfoodfarm.com

Freitas Farm, 32 Wood Street, Middleborough, MA. Phone: 508-947-6521. Sustainable Farm that does not use chemicals on their produce (with a few exceptions like their peaches). Freitas is a large, local farm that is a frequent vendor at farmers markets around the south shore. This farm grows apples, strawberries, carrots, lettuce, peas, pumpkins, beans, squash, tomatoes, etc. Find them at the following farmers markets: Brockton, Carver, Dedham, Hingham, Kingston, Marshfield, Natick, Randolph, Sandwich, and Quincy farmers markets. https://www.facebook.com/FreitasFarm/

Fresh Meadows, 43 North Main St., Carver, MA. Phone: 508-866-7136. Organic Farm. This farm grows organic cranberries, fresh cranberries are available October through December while supplies last, and they sell out fast. Frozen organic cranberries are available year-round while supplies last. Farm stand at 39 North Main Street aka Rt. 58 is open weekends in October, weather permitting noon to 5:00 PM. Find them at the following farmers markets: Plymouth Farmers Market at Plimoth Plantation. http://freshmeadowscranberries.com

Greenway Farm, 48 Marion Drive, Kingston, MA 02364. Phone: 781-201-0646. Sustainable Farm. CSA available. This farm grows lettuce, edible flowers, herbs, microgreens, and eggs. Find them at the following farmers markets: Kingston Farmers Market. https://squareup.com/store/greenwayfarmkingston

Heart Beets Farm, 181 Bayview Ave., Berkley, MA. Phone: 508-822-6919. Certified Organic Farm. This farm grows tomatoes, lettuce, potatoes, squash, peppers, onions, carrots, etc. CSA Available. Farm Stand "honesty stand" open Saturday's 9:00 AM to 5:00 PM seasonally from May to November. Farm stand is located in the bottom of the Red Barn on their farm. They sell what they grow and do not buy from other farms. Find them at the following farmers markets: Taunton and Somerset open air market. https://www.heartbeetsfarm.com/

Hillside Mushrooms, Colebrook Rd, Little Compton, RI. Phone: 401-486-0796. Sustainable Farm. This farm grows gourmet mushrooms including; Golden Oyster, Nameko, King Oyster, Blue Oyster, Lion's Mane, Shiitake Mushrooms etc. Find them at the following farmers markets: Marshfield Fair Farmers Market and the Plymouth Farmers Market. https://www.facebook.com/hillsidemushroomsri/

Holly Hill Farm, 236 Jerusalem Road, Cohasset MA 02025. Phone: 781-383-1455. Organic Farm. This farm grows flowers, herbs, seedlings, beans (green), beets (sugar), kale, potatoes, tomatoes, etc. Farm stand is open Saturday & Sunday 10:00 AM -4:00 PM May through December. Find them at the following farmers markets: Cohasset and Scituate. http://www.hollyhillfarm.org/

Ichabod Flat Oysters, Plymouth, MA. Sustainably raised, hand harvested oysters. https://www.ichabodflat.com/

Indian Cove Aquaculture, Onset, MA 02558. Phone: 508-776-2542. Sustainable Farm. Farm raised oysters and quahogs grown in the Wareham, Buzzards Bay and Cape Cod Canal area waters. Find them at the Wareham Oyster Festival. http://indiancoveaquaculture.com/

Island Creek Oysters, 296 Parks Street, Duxbury, MA 02332. Phone: 781-934-2028. Sustainable Farm. This farm grows oysters in Duxbury Bay. Sometimes they might have razor clams, Nantucket bay scallops, or whelks. Duxbury retail store is open Sunday and Monday noon -5:00 PM, Tuesday through Saturday 10:00 AM - 6:00 PM. http://www.islandcreekoysters.com/

Jenney Grist Mill Museum, 48 Summer Street, Plymouth, MA 02360. Phone: 508-747-4544. Organic and Sustainable Farm. Organic and ground cornmeal, sampe, rye flour. The Museum shop is open Monday thru Saturday 9:00 AM -5:00 PM, closed Sundays. They grind on Friday and Saturday afternoons from 1:00 PM -3:00 PM. Farm products can be found at The Indoor Plymouth Farmers Market at Plimoth Plantation. https://www.plimoth.com/collections/plimoth-grist-mill

Lane Gardens, Rte. 138, 1758 Somerset Avenue, Dighton, MA 02715. Certified Naturally Grown. They grow lettuce, strawberries, chard, broccoli, zucchini, tomatoes, etc. Find them at the following farmers markets: Randolph and Stoughton. http://www.lanegardens.org/ https://www.facebook.com/lane.gardens.7

Langwater Farm, Stone Soup LLC, 209 Washington St. route 138, North Easton, MA 02356. Phone: 508- 205-9665. USDA Organic Farm. This farm grows beans, corn, peaches, peppers, potatoes, spinach, strawberries, tomatoes, squash, etc. Farm Boxes available. Farm stand is open Tuesdays through Sundays 10:00 AM -6:00 PM, closed Mondays. Find them at the following farmers markets: Attleboro, Braintree Town Hall, Pawtucket Wintertime Farmers Market, and the Original Easton Farmers Market. https://langwaterfarm.com

Lipinski's Farm, 19 Franklin St., Hanson, MA 02333. Phone: 781-293-3440. This is a sustainable and local farm that uses minimal pesticides on most of their crops. But, some crops do get sprayed such as their corn. Their farm stand is open daily during the season from 9:30 AM to 6:30 PM. Find them at the following farmers markets: South Weymouth. http://lipinskifarm.com/

Natick Community Organic Farm, 117 Eliot Street, Natick MA 01760. Phone: 508-655-2204. Organic Farm. This farm produces maple syrup, berries, flowers, herbs, seedlings, vegetables, celery, and wool from their sheep. CSA available. The Farm land is open to the public every day. Farm stand is a self-serve, honor-system, market stand open during daylight hours in the spring, summer and fall, cash or check only. Find them at the following farmers markets: Natick Farmers Market. https://www.natickfarm.org

Nest and Song Farm, 3 Stone Fruit Lane, Westport, MA 02790. Phone: 781-426-1382. Sustainable Farm. This farm grows vegetables, fruit, eggs and meat, lettuce, peppers, potatoes, strawberries, sweet potatoes, etc. Farm Shares available. Find them at the following farmers markets: Hope & Main Schoolyard Market in Warren, RI from June to October 10:00 AM -2:00 PM. http://www.nestandsongfarm.com/

Norwell Farms, 4 Jacobs Lane, Norwell, MA 02061. Organic Farm. Non-profit, community Farm. This farm grows organic vegetables, meat and flowers. CSA available. Organic vegetable, meat, and flower shares are available. Norwell Farms partners with Freedom Food Farm and Cross Street Flower Farm. Farm stand is open for CSA pick up on Thursdays 3:00 PM -7:00 PM and Saturday 9:00 AM -noon. http://www.norwellfarms.org/

Not Enough Acres Farms, 107 Sesuit Neck Rd., East Dennis, MA 02641. Phone: 508-737-3446. Certified Naturally grown Farm. Farm stand is open daily, year-round, sun up to sun down. Find them at the Harwich Farmers Market.

Oakdale Farm, 61 Wheaton Ave., Rehoboth, MA. Phone: 508-336-7681. Partially organic and the rest is sustainably farmed using IPM. The farm has a shop, hayrides, and corn maze. Find them at the following farmers markets: Easton and Scituate. https://www.facebook.com/Oakdale-Farms-Country-Barn-and-Garden-Shop-103128933640/

Peachtree Circle Farm, 881 Palmer Ave., Falmouth, MA 02543. Organic Farm. Peachtree Circle Farm follows organic farming practices, while not certified as an organic farm. This farm grows raspberries, blackberries, lavender, apples, peaches, pears, arugula, beets, garlic, lettuce, peppers, pineapple tomatillos, potatoes, squash, and tomatoes. CSA available. Find them at the following farmers markets: Falmouth Farmers Market- summer at Peg Noonan Park and winters at Mahoney's. https://www.peachtreecirclefarm.com/

Plato's Harvest, Middleboro, MA. Organic farm. This 3-acre farm grows Flowers, Herbs, Seed Crops, Seedlings, and Vegetables. Find them at the following farmers markets: Plymouth Farmers Market. https://www.facebook.com/platosharvest/

R & C Farms-Simons Greenhouse, Rte. 123, 124 Cornet Stetson Road, Scituate, MA 02066. Telephone: 781-545-6502. Sustainable Farm. They use little to no pesticides and only when necessary. This farm grows corn, zucchini, lettuce, cucumbers, onions, potatoes, peppers, beets, beans, berries, tomatoes, eggplant, etc. They partner with the Belkin Family Lookout Farm of Natick for some of their fruits and apples. CSA available. Farm stand and greenhouse open daily 9:00 AM -6:00 PM. http://www.randcfarms-simons.com/

RI Mushroom Co., 141 Fairgrounds Rd., West Kingston, RI 02892. Phone: 401-250-3999. Sustainable Farm. This farm grows several varieties of mushroom including Blue Oyster, Crimini, Golden Oyster, King Oyster, Maitake, Portobello, and Pioppino. Find them at the following farmers markets: Marshfield Fair, and RI markets; Pawtucket Wintertime Market, Hope Street Market, Coastal Growers Market, South Kingston Market, Aquidneck Growers Market, Mount Hope Market, and Richmond Market. http://www.rimushrooms.com/

River Street Garden, Halifax, MA. Phone: 781-294-0589. Organic Farm. We are a small family run organic grower who focuses on vegetables and herbs. Find them at the following farmers markets: Marshfield Fair Farmers Market. https://www.facebook.com/riverstreet.gardens/

Robbins Trout Farm, West Wareham, MA. Phone: 508-294-1796. Sustainable Farm. This farm raises trout in the wild, in spring fed water. Find them at the following farmers markets: Mattapoisett. Also available at a few select markets and restaurants. Check their website for up-to-date information. http://robbinstroutfarm.com/Home_Page.html

Round The Bend Farm, 92 Allen's Neck Road, South Dartmouth, MA 02748. Phone: 508-938-5127. Sustainable Farm. Chemical-free produce, local honey, grass-fed meat. Open farm days are every third Saturday from 10:00 AM -5:00 PM. www.roundthebendfarm.org.

Russell Orchards, 143 Argilla Rd., Ipswich, MA. Phone: 978-356-5366. Sustainable Farm. Naturally Grown produce using Integrated Pest Management. PYO available. This farm grows cherries, strawberries, raspberries, currants, blueberries, blackberries, apples, celery, garlic scapes, kale, lavender, leeks, potatoes, spinach, tomatillos, apricots, cherries, currants, elderberries-in August, gooseberries, grapes, jostaberries, nectarines, peaches, pears, plums, etc. They also have a Winery that makes fruit wines and a bakery. Wine tastings are Friday to Sunday from noon to 5:00 PM. Farm Store is open seasonally 9:00 AM-6:00 PM daily. Always check their website for the most up-to-date information. https://www.russellorchards.com/

Sauchuk Farm, 53 Palmer Road (Route 58), Plympton, MA. Phone: 781-585-1522. Sustainable Farm. This farm uses organic and sustainable practices including IPM. This farm grows corn, strawberries, blueberries, lettuce, etc. CSA available. PYO available. Corn Maze at 200 Center Street in Plympton is open weekends from late September to early November. There is plenty to do at the corn maze and pumpkin patch including hay wagon rides, corn cannon game, barnyard basketball game, and plenty of other activities and games for adults and children. Farm Stand is open daily from 9:00AM to 6:00 PM. Sauchuck farm grows over eighty percent of the products sold at the farm stand. http://www.sauchukfarm.com/

Second Nature Farm, 97 Crane St., Norton, MA. Phone: 774-266-0431. Sustainable Farm. Certified Naturally Grown Farm. They farm without chemicals or pesticides. This farm grows spinach, beans, beets, celery, garlic, kale, lettuce, potatoes, peppers, strawberries, squash, tomatoes, etc. CSA available. Find them at the following farmers markets: Braintree and Hingham Farmers Market from May-November.
https://www.secondnaturefarm.com/

Silverbrook Farms, 592 Chase Rd Dartmouth, MA 02747. Sustainable Farm. This farm grows kale, lettuce, shitake mushrooms, free range eggs, strawberries, peas, duck eggs, blueberries, blue oyster mushrooms, corn, beets, peaches, apples, peppers, tomatoes and potatoes. CSA available. Farmstand open seasonally noon-6:00 PM. Find them at the following farmers markets: Falmouth, Dartmouth, Provincetown, and SoWa Open Market.
http://www.silverbrookdartmouth.com/

Skinny Dip Farm, 1603 Main Road, Westport, MA. Phone: 401-592-0237. Certified Organic Farm. This farm grows arugula, spinach, beans, beets, broccoli, Brussels sprouts, cabbage, carrots, celeriac, chard, cucumbers, edamame, eggplant, fennel, kale, kohlrabi, leeks, lettuce (8 varieties), Napa cabbage, onions (6 varieties), parsnips, peas (sugar snap), peppers (sweet and hot specialty varieties), popcorn, potatoes (new and fingerling), radishes, scallions, shallots, summer squash, tomatoes (including about 15 different heirlooms), cherry tomatoes, turnips, winter squash, etc. Find them at the following farmers markets: Plymouth Farmers Market at

Plimoth Plantation, Westport, and Falmouth.
https://m.facebook.com/skinny.farm/,
http://skinnydipfarm.blogspot.com/

Skymeadow Orchards, Scituate, MA. Phone: 781-545-9418. Sustainable Farm. This farm grows six varieties of pesticide-free Asian pears. Asian pears are ready around late September until November. Find them at the following farmers markets: The Indoor Plymouth Farmers Market at Plimoth Plantation and Marshfield Fair Farmers Market. Always check the Plymouth/Marshfield Farmers Market Facebook or website for the most up-to-date information.

Tuck-A-Way-Farm, 2 Barkley Way, Harwich, Ma. Phone: 508-237-3515. Sustainable Farm. No GMO seeds and organic seeds whenever possible. This farm grows apples, tomatoes, corn, potatoes, spinach, lettuce, kale, strawberries, honey, eggs, maple syrup etc. Roadside Stand in Harwich. Find them at the following farmers markets: Harwich and Chatham.
http://www.tuckawayfarmofharwich.com/

Twelve Moon Farm, 18 Capen St., Milton, MA 02186. Organic Farm. This farm grows vegetables, herbs, flowers, seedlings, organic produce, greens and heirloom vegetables. Find them at the following farmers markets: Milton Farmers Market. Check their website or Instagram for the most up-to-date information.
https://twelvemoonfarm.com/

Ward's Berry Farm, 614 South Main Street, Sharon, MA. Phone: 781-784-3600. Sustainable Farm. This farm grows some organic crops but otherwise practices sustainable farming methods using IPM and limited pesticides. PYO available. This farm grows strawberries, blueberries, pumpkins, currants, gooseberries, melons, peaches, apricots, cherries, broccoli, lettuce, spinach, onions, peppers, potatoes, squash, tomatoes, corn, eggplant, grapes etc. CSA and Farm Boxes available. Farm Store open year-round, weekdays 9:00 AM to 7:00 PM, weekends 9:00 AM-6:00 PM. The produce in the store is clearly labelled by origin on each item. They sell sandwiches, salads, baked goods, and smoothies, along with local and artisanal products in the store. http://www.wardsberryfarm.com/FARM.html

Web of Life Farm, 71 Silva Street, Carver, MA 02330. Phone: 508-866-7712. Organic and Sustainable Farm. This farm grows peppers (sweet bell), tomatoes, heritage and heirloom varieties of vegetables, apples, grapes, etc. They also raise and sell poultry and turkeys, honey and eggs. Farm Boxes available. Find them at the following farmers markets: The Indoor Plymouth Farmers Market at Plimoth Plantation and Hingham Farmers Market. https://www.weboflifefarm.com/

West Elm Farm, 65 West Elm Street, Pembroke, MA. Phone: 617-435-3372. Sustainable Farm. This small eco-farm produces wool products, goat's milk & lanolin soap, hand balm, organic chicken, farm raised rabbit meat & duck eggs. Whole freezer lambs are available in the Fall (September & October). Can be found at Marshfield Fair Farmers Market. http://www.westelmfarm.com/

White Barn Farm, 458 South Street, Wrentham, MA 02093. Phone: 774-210-0359. Organic Farm. This farm grows beets, lettuce, spinach, carrots, cucumbers, tomatoes, peppers, etc. Weekly CSA available. Farm stand spring hours (May to June) Friday 10:00 AM -6:00 PM, weekends 10:00 AM -4:00 PM. Summer hours (June through October) are Tuesday through Friday, 10:00 AM -6:00 PM, weekends, 10:00 AM -4:00 PM. Fall hours in the white barn from November through December, Friday 10:00 AM -6:00 PM and weekends, 10:00 AM -4:00 PM. The farm stand sells its own produce, seedlings, and flowers. They also sell local honey, maple syrup, mushrooms, pasture raised meat, eggs, etc. http://whitebarnfarm.org/

Winters Farm, 4 Tremont St, Rehoboth, MA. Phone: 508-272-2095. Sustainable Farm. This farm raises grass fed beef, pastured pork, and pastured chicken eggs. Check out their Facebook page for the most up-to-date information. https://www.facebook.com/Winters-Farm-762965210491033/.

HONORABLE MENTION FARMS

These farms may or may not be organic or use sustainable farming methods but they are worth mention due to their high quality produce, community involvement, amenities, unique produce, or popularity. The top honorable mention farms in and around the South Shore, include (but are not limited to):

Blueberry Farm, The. 698 West Washington St., Hanson, MA 02341. Phone: 781-447-1584. Local Farm. This farm grows blueberries. This is a seasonal PYO farm open mid-July through August, daily-depending upon weather and crop yield. Check their Facebook page or call ahead for hours. https://www.facebook.com/The-Blueberry-Farm-129207739514/

Breezy Knoll Farm, Rehoboth, MA. This farm sells tomatoes, squashes, potatoes, zucchini, etc. Find them at Taunton Farmers market.

Cape Cod Lavender Farm, off Weston Woods Road, Harwich, MA. Phone: 508-432-8397. Fields of lavender plants on twelve secluded acres surrounded by seventy-five acres of conservation land and walking trails. Harvest season is mid-June to mid-July. They have a farm store with an assortment of lavender soaps, salves, lotions, candles, etc. https://www.capecodlavenderfarm.com/

Cape Cod Winery, 4 Oxbow Rd, East Falmouth, MA 02536. Phone: 508-457-5592. The grapes are grown right there and both tastings and tours are available. https://capecodwinery.com/

Carolyn's Sakonnet Vineyard, 162 W Main Rd, Little Compton, RI 02837. Phone: 401-635-8486. The grapes are grown right there and both tastings and tours are available. Check out all the local wineries on the coastal wine trail. https://www.sakonnetwine.com/

Connors Farm, 30 Valley Road (Rt. 35), Danvers, Massachusetts 01923. Not organic or super local but a farm worth mentioning because of its events and amenities. With an entrance fee this farm offers a haunted farm, flashlight maze, a singles night, a farm stand, PYO strawberries, peaches, pumpkins, etc. Opens June 15th thru the fall. Check their website or Facebook page for prices and what is available each week. https://www.connorsfarm.com/

Coutinho Farm, Berkley, MA. Phone: 508-930-6532. This farm grows apples, berries, cantaloupe, figs, grapes, melons, peaches, pears, plums, quince, watermelons, eggplant, potatoes, tomatoes, zucchini, etc. Find them at the Fall River and Taunton Farmer's Market.

Crescent Ridge Dairy, 355 Bay Road, Sharon, MA 02067. Phone: 781-784-2740. This farm makes their own milk, cream, butter and ice cream from their farm. They deliver to area residents. They also sell their own grass-fed farm raised meat. They partner with local farms and offer produce boxes and over 100 locally sourced products with your delivery. https://crescentridge.deliverybizpro.com/home.php

Hanson Farm, 600 Pleasant St (rte. 104), Bridgewater, MA. Phone: 508-697-4003. This farm grows and sells sweet corn, vegetables, eggs and honey. They partner with CN Smith farm for some of their fruit including apples, nectarines, and peaches. Sugar Hill Dairy, an ice cream store is next to their farm stand. The farm stand is open 8:00 AM to 6:00 PM daily, May through December. http://www.hansonfarm.com/

Hornstra Farms, 246 Prospect Street, Norwell, MA 02061. Phone: 781-749-1222. This farm makes their own milk, cream, butter and ice cream from their farm with minimal pasteurization. They deliver to area residents and milk can be ordered in either plastic or milk bottles. They also have a store where they sell their products plus other local quality items and ice cream cones. Farm store in Norwell is open daily from 10:00 AM -8:00 PM. The Ice Cream Dairy Bar is open daily from noon to 8:00 PM. http://hornstrafarms.com/

Just Right Farm, 140 Palmer Rd, Plympton, MA 02367. RESERVATIONS 781-936-5330. A farm-to-table restaurant. Enjoy a purely local produce and protein prix fixe dinner in the farm's screen house. They have Twilight Garden Parties on selected Thursdays from June to September from 6:00 PM -8:00 PM at around $85 per person. Eat dinner at the Chef's table for around $175 per person for five courses. Check out their website for more information and to make reservations. http://justrightfarm.com/

Lally Farms, Hanover, MA 02339. Phone: 781-878-4014. Family owned farm in Hanover that sells their eggs, butter, cheese and meats to local grocery markets. They partner with milk delivery companies in the area such as Hornstra Farms and Crescent Ridge. https://www.lallyfarms.com/

Lanni Orchards, Rt. 13, 294 Chase Rd, Lunenburg, Massachusetts 01462. Phone: 978-582-6246. This farm is not on the South Shore but can be found at local farmer's markets. This is a sustainable farm that practices Integrated Pest Management, doesn't spray their berries and uses the least amount of pesticides on the rest of their crops. They grow strawberries, asparagus, rhubarb, lettuce, garlic, grapes, apples, raspberries, pumpkins, tomatoes, etc. Find them at the following farmers markets: South Weymouth. www.facebook.com/LanniOrchards/

Littles Creek Farm, Marshfield, MA 02050. Phone: 781-837-8727. Organic and sustainable Farm. This farm grows vegetables. Find them at the following farmers markets: Marshfield Fair Farmers Market.

Miami Fruit, 7900 SW 40th St, Miami, FL 33155. Organic Farm and Sustainable Farm. Although this is not a local farm it is a good place to order organic fruit in the winter. This farm grows avocados, bananas, cocoa nibs, coconuts, exotic fruit, etc. Most of the fruits are USDA organic and/or sustainably farmed. They sell their fruit online and ship to Massachusetts. They pick their fruit on Mondays and ship on Tuesdays. Check their website for fruit readiness and prices. https://miamifruit.org/

Mounce Farm, 481 Union St., Marshfield, MA. PYO apples in September. Look for the sign on Union Street.

Plymouth Bay Winery, 114 Water St, Plymouth, MA 02360. Phone: 508-746-2100. Wines produced from locally grown, native grapes and berries. Wine made in Plymouth, MA. http://plymouthbaywinery.com/

Queen Bee Honey Products, 201 Dwelley Street, Pembroke, MA 02359. Telephone 781-829-8817. All natural honey products for healthy skin, body and mind. They use their own honey from their farm in Pembroke, MA. Products can be found in local markets and farmers markets. http://queenbeehoney.com

Rye Tavern, 517 Old Sandwich Rd, Plymouth, MA 02360. Phone: 508-591-7515. Not a farm but a farm-to-table restaurant. They use produce and other ingredients from local and sustainable farms. Open all week starting at 5:00 PM for dinner (bar opens at 4:00 PM) and Saturday and Sunday Brunch from 11:00 AM to 2:00 PM. Outdoor Patio is open in the spring and summer. www.ryetavern.com

South Shore Organics. Delivery of organic or locally and sustainable produce and meats to the South Shore area. They partner with local farmers to bring you the freshest, local, produce on the South Shore. They work with farms such as; Allen Farms, Aquidneck Farms, Baffoni's Poultry, Barden Family Orchard, Brown Boar Farm, Colchester Neighborhood Farm, Feather Brook Farm, Freedom Food Farm, Langwater Farm, Plato's Harvest, and many more. Check out their website to learn more; https://southshoreorganics.deliverybizpro.com/p-40-how-it-works-subpage.html

The Farmer's Daughter, 122 Main St., Easton, MA 02356. Phone: 508-297-0286. Not a farm but a farm-to-table restaurant. They use produce and other ingredients from local and sustainable farms. Open Tuesday-Friday (Closed Mondays) 8:00 AM -2:00 PM. Saturday and Sunday 7:00 AM -3:00 PM. They are open for dinner on Thursday, Friday, and Saturday from 6:00 PM-11:00 PM.

Tree-Berry Farm, 135 Cornet Stetson Rd, Scituate, MA 02066. Phone 781-545-7750. They grow and sell blueberries and Christmas Trees. Blueberry season is late July through August. Hours are 7:00 AM to 1:00 PM during the season depending upon weather. http://www.treeberryfarm.com/

Truro Vineyards, 11 Shore Rd, North Truro, MA 02652. Phone: 508-487-6200. This is a sustainable vineyard on the Cape Cod shoreline. The grapes are grown right there and both tastings and tours are available. Open seven days Monday-Saturday 11:00 AM -5:00 PM; Sunday noon-5:00 PM. https://trurovineyardsofcapecod.com/

Weir River Farm Market, 140 Turkey Hill Ln, Hingham, MA 02043. This farm offers non-certified organically grown produce. They can be found at the Hingham Farmers Market. https://www.facebook.com/weirriverfarm/

Westport Rivers Vineyard, 417 Hixbridge Rd, Westport, MA 02790. Phone: 508-636-3423. "The Russell's founded both Buzzards Bay Brewing and Westport Rivers Winery upon this deep regard for local agriculture and education. As of 2012, the Russell Family has permanently preserved 400 acres of working farmland and forest." The grapes are grown right there and both tastings and tours are available. Check out other wineries on the coastal wine trail. http://www.westportrivers.com

White Gate Gardens, 687 Union Street, Duxbury, MA. Sustainable Farm. This farm grows tomatoes, squash, radishes, garlic, onions, sunflowers, etc. The farm stand [Honesty Stand] open May thru October with seasonal produce only.

FARM MAP

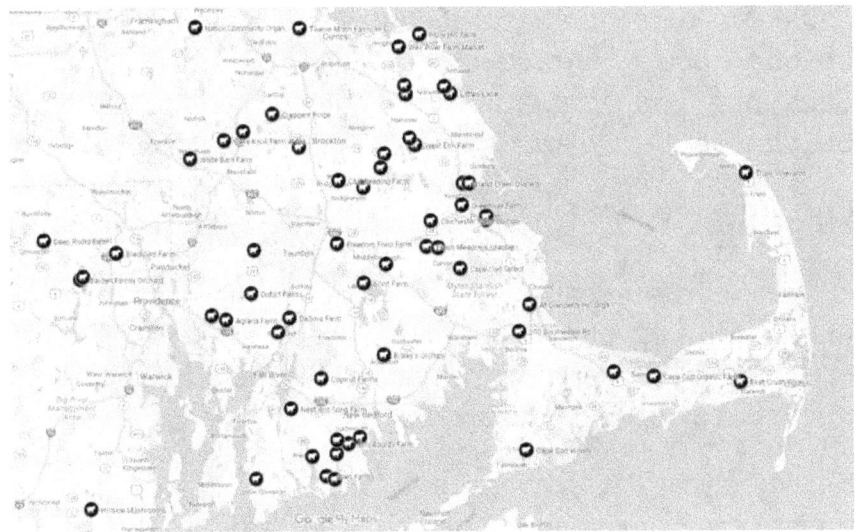

FARMERS MARKETS

It's nearly impossible to get to all the farms of your choice but you might be able to buy from many of them at the same place and same time. Farmers markets are a great way to shop in one spot for all your farm-fresh produce.

The farmer market bounty is usually sparse during May and early June. The best months with a guaranteed abundant bounty of produce are July and August. September and October are good too but it all depends on the weather that year.

Check the produce availability chart to find out what is in season each week before heading to the farmers market. Or, look at the website or Facebook page of your farmers market for a list of vendors and available produce. If you can't get to the market consider downloading a farmers market app such as, *Market2Day*.

Be aware that dates, times, and locations change from time to time so call ahead before heading out to the farmers market. Whether you are home or on vacation make sure to check out the *MassGrown Map* on the Mass.gov website for the most up-to-date information on farmers markets in your area, http://www.mass.gov/agr/massgrown/

Acushnet Farmers Market. Stone Bridge Farm, 186 Leonard St., Acushnet, MA 02743. Saturday, 10:00 AM - 2:00 PM. Market is open from June to September. http://acushnetfarmersmarket.com/

Andover Farmers Market. 97 Main St.-Andover Center for History and Culture, Andover, MA 01810. Saturday, 10:00 AM - 2:00 PM. Market is open from June to October. http://andoverhistoryandculture.org/farmers-market

Attleboro Farmers Market. O'Connell Field at Capron Park, 201 County Street, Attleboro, MA 02703. Saturday, 9:00 AM - 1:00 PM. Market is open from June to October. http://attleborofarmersmarket.com

Braintree Farmers Market. Town Hall, 1 JFK Memorial Drive, Braintree, MA. Saturday, 9:00 AM – 1:00 PM. Market is open from June to October. Special indoor Thanksgiving Market in November. Vendors: Langwater Farm, DaSilva Farm, Foxboro Cheese and Veal, Fresh Catch, Vermont Syrup Company, J.H. Beaulieu Livestock and Produce Farm, Second Nature Farm. www.BraintreeFarmersMarket.org

Brewster Farmers Market. Windmill Village, 51 Drummer Boy Road, Brewster, MA. Sunday, 9:00 AM-1:00 PM. Market is open from June to September. WIC & Senior Coupons Accepted EBT-SNAP Accepted. http://www.brewsterhistoricalsociety.org/farmers-market/

Bridgewater West Farmers Market. First Church of West Bridgewater, 29 Howard Street, West Bridgewater, MA. Tuesdays, 4:00 PM to 7:00 PM. Select Dates in June, August and November, check website or Facebook page. https://www.facebook.com/WBFarmersMarket/

Brockton Fairgrounds Farmers Market. Brockton Fairgrounds, 600 Belmont St., Brockton, MA 02301. Saturday, 9:00 AM - 12:00 PM. Market is open from July to October. WIC & Senior Coupons Accepted. EBT-SNAP Accepted.

Brockton Farmers Market. City Hall Plaza, 45 School Street, Brockton, MA 02301. Friday 10:00 AM - 2:00 PM. Market is open from July to October. WIC & Senior Coupons Accepted and EBT-SNAP Accepted.

Carver Farmers Market. Shurtleff Park, across from Town Hall, Rt. 58, 108 Main Street, Carver, MA 02330. Sunday, Noon - 4:00 PM. Market is open from June to October. WIC & Senior Coupons Accepted. SNAP-EBT Accepted with select vendors only. https://www.facebook.com/pages/Carver-Farmers-Market/167244363347318

Chatham Farmers Market. 1652 Main Street, Local Color and Ocean State Job Lot Parking Lot, South Chatham, MA 02659. Tuesday, 3:00 PM - 6:00 PM. Market is open from May to October. WIC & Senior Coupons Accepted. Vendors: Allen Farms, Westminster Meats, Tuck-A-Way-Farm, Not Enough Acres Farm.

https://www.facebook.com/Chatham-Farmers-Market-100705810022669/

Cohasset Farmers Market. Historic Cohasset Common, 27 S Main St, Cohasset, MA 02025. Thursday, 2:00 PM – 6:00 PM. Market is open from June to October. Vendors: Cretinon's Farm Stand, Holly Hill Farm. www.cohassetfarmersmarket.com

Dartmouth Farmers Market. St. Mary's Parish, 789 Dartmouth Street, Dartmouth, MA. Friday, 1:00 PM – 6:00 PM. Market is open from June to October. Vendors: Apponagansett Farm (sustainable), Copicut Farms, Silk Tree Farm, Silverbrook Farms (sustainable). http://www.dartmouthfarmersmarket.com/

Easton Summer Farmers Market aka Original Easton Farmers Market. 591 Depot St, North Easton, MA 02356. Saturday, 10:00 AM - 2:00 PM. Market is open from May to October. WIC & Senior Coupons Accepted. EBT-SNAP Accepted. Vendors: Langwater Farms, Foxboro Cheese Co, Rosie Bud honey farm of Wrentham, Oakdale Farm, etc. http://www.easton.ma.us/boards_and_committees/agricultural_commission/click_here.php

Easton Farmers Market. Marketplace at Simpson Spring, 719 Washington Street, Easton, MA. Saturday, 10:00 AM -2:00 PM. Year-Round Market. https://www.simpsonspring.com/saturday-market

Easton Winter Farmers Market. Oakes Ames Memorial Hall, 3 Barrows St. Easton, MA. Saturdays, 10:00 AM - 2:00 PM. Market is open from November through May. Vendors: Langwater Farms, Foxboro Cheese Co. http://www.easton.ma.us/boards_and_committees/agricu ltural_commission/click_here.php

Falmouth Summer Farmers Market. Marine Park overlooking Falmouth Harbor, 180 Scranton Ave, Falmouth, MA 02540. Thursday, noon-6:00 PM. Market is open from May thru October. Vendors: Silverbrook Farms, Peachtree Circle Farm, and Allen Farms Organics. http://www.falmouthfarmersmarket.org/

Falmouth Winter Farmers Market. at Mahoney's Garden Center, 958 E Falmouth Hwy, East Falmouth, MA 02536. Saturdays, 10:00 AM -3:00 PM. Market is open from around November thru April. Vendors: Silverbrook Farms, Peachtree Circle Farm, Allen Farms Organics. http://www.falmouthfarmersmarket.org/

Harwich Farmers Market. 80 Parallel St,-Harwich Historical Society, Rt. 39, Harwich , MA 02645. Thursday, 3:00 PM - 6:00 PM. Market is open from June to October. WIC & Senior Coupons Accepted. Vendors: Not Enough Acres Farm. http://harwichfarmersmarket.org/

Hingham Summer Farmers Market. Hingham Bathing Beach Parking lot, Route 3A, 96 Otis Street, Hingham, MA, 02043. Saturday, 10:00 AM – 2:00 PM. Market is open from May to November. Rain or shine. Vendors:

Vermont Syrup, Second Nature Farm, Copicut Farms, Narragansett Creamery, Freitas Farm, etc. www.HinghamFarmersMarket.org

Hingham Winter Farmers Market. Second Parish Church, 685 Main Street, Hingham MA, 02043. Second and fourth Saturday, 10:00 AM to 1:00 PM. Market is open from January thru March. Vendors: Copicut Farms, Narragansett Creamery, Freitas Farm, etc. http://hinghamfarmersmarket.org/

Holbrook Farmers Market. Union Street Lanes bowling alley parking lot, 231 Union St., Holbrook, MA 02343. Saturday, 9:00 AM - 2:00 PM. Market is open from June to Mid-October. WIC & Senior Coupons Accepted. https://www.facebook.com/HolbrookFarmersMarket

Hyannis Summer Farmers Market. 1336 Phinney's Lane-Cape Cod Beer, HYANNIS, MA 02601. Friday, 3:00 PM - 6:00 PM. Market is open from late May to late September. WIC & Senior Coupons Accepted. Vendors: CapeAbilitis Farm. http://capecodbeer.com/farmersmarketmeetshappyhour/

Hyannis Winter Farmers Market. A Very Merry Market at Cape Cod Beer. 1336 Phinnys Lane, Hyannis MA. Saturdays, 11:00 AM-4:00 PM. Market is open from November through December. https://capecodbeer.com/event/merry-market-pop-up-cape-cod/2018-12-22/

Kingston Farmers Market (new market!). 101 Kingston Collection Way, Kingston, MA 02364. Sunday, 10:00 AM – 2:00 PM. First Sunday of the month only. Market is open from June to October. Vendors: Greenway Farm, Bogside Acres, Boston Bee Co., etc. https://www.farmersmarketkingston.com/

Kingston's Stonecroft Place Farmers Market (new market). At Indian Pond Estates, 431 Country Club Way, Kingston, MA 02364. Last Tuesday of each month, 3:00 PM-6:00 PM. Market is open from May through October. https://www.facebook.com/StonecroftPlaceFarmersMarket

Marshfield Summer Farmers Market. Marshfield Fairgrounds, Rt. 3A, 140 Main Street, Marshfield, MA. Friday, 2:00 PM – 6:00 PM. Market is open from June to October. NOTE: market will be held Friday, 2:00 PM – 6:00 PM at the town hall green during the Marshfield Fair dates. Vendors: Brown Boar Farm, DaSilva, Foxboro Cheese, Hillside Mushrooms, Littles Creek Farm, Skymeadow Orchards, West Elm Farm. http://marshfieldfair.org/farmers-market/

Marshfield Winter Farmers Market. Under the Grandstand, Marshfield Fairgrounds, Rt. 3A, 140 Main Street, Marshfield, MA 02050. Third Saturday of the Month, 10:00 AM – 2:00 PM. Market is open from November to May. SNAP/EBT accepted. http://marshfieldfair.org/farmers-market/

Mattapoisett Farmers Market aka Old-Rochester-Tri-Town Farmers Market. Old Rochester Regional Junior High School, 135 Marion Road, Mattapoisett, MA. Tuesday, 3:00 PM -6:00 PM. Market is open from June to October. Vendors: Cervelli's Farm, Weatherlow Farms, Skinny Dip Farm, etc. http://rfmarket.blogspot.com/

Middleboro Farmers Market. Oliver Mill Park, Route 44 East, 8 Nemasket Street, Middleboro, MA 02346. Saturday, 10:00 AM - 2:00 PM. Market is open from June to October. WIC & Senior Coupons Accepted. Vendors: Freitas Farm, M & O Farms, Sweetbrier Farms, etc. http://www.middleboroughfarmersmarket.com/

Middleborough Farmers Market aka Farmers' Market of Middleboro. 225 Wood Street, Middleboro, Massachusetts 02346. Saturday 9:30 AM-1:00 PM. Market is open from June to October. EBT and HIP accepted. www.facebook.com/FarmersMarketofMiddleborough/

Milton Farmers Market. Milton Village, Wharf Street, Milton, MA. Thursdays, 1:00 PM -6:00 PM. Market is open from June through October. Vendors: Copicut Farm, Foxboro Cheese, E. L. Silvia Farms, Twelve Moon Farm, etc. http://www.miltonmassfarmersmarket.org/

Mount Hope Farm Indoor Farmers Market. The Barn at Mount Hope Farm, 250 Metacom Avenue, Bristol, RI 02809. Saturdays, 9:00 AM-12:30 PM year-round. Vendors: Barden Family Orchard, Foxboro Cheese, Maplewood Farm, RI Mushroom Co., Roots Farm, etc., http://www.mounthopefarm.org/community-programs/farmers-market

Natick Farmers Market. Natick Common or at the Common Street Spirituality Center, 13 Common St, Natick, MA 01760. Saturday, 9:00 AM -1:00 PM year-round. Vendors: Narragansett Creamery, Natick Community Organic Farm, Nicewicz Orchards, Oakdale Farms, organic, Wildwood Mushrooms of Sutton. http://www.natickfarmersmarket.com/

New Bedford Farmers Market. Clasky Common Park, 1118 Pleasant St., New Bedford, MA. Saturday 10:00 AM - 2:00 PM. Market is open from June to October. Free Parking. Vendors: Al's Backwoods Berrie Co., Bergies Seafood, Noquochoke orchards, Peets Farm, Buzzards Bay Bee Company, LLC, Kyler's Catch Seafood Market, Brix Bounty Farm, Stony Creek Farm and grass-fed beef, Wyandotte Farm, etc. https://coastalfoodshed.org/new-bedford-farmersmarkets. https://www.facebook.com/newbedfordfarmersmarket/

New Bedford Farmers Market. Brooklawn Park, 1997 Acushnet Ave, New Bedford, MA 02745 (near the duck pond on the Acushnet Ave side). Mondays, 2:00 PM -6:00 PM. Market is open from June to October. Free Parking. www.facebook.com/newbedfordfarmersmarket/

New Bedford Farmers Market. Custom House Square, 21 Barkers Ln, New Bedford, MA 02740. Thursday's 2:00 PM -6:00 PM. Market is open from June to October. Free 30 Minute parking and metered parking. www.facebook.com/newbedfordfarmersmarket/

New Bedford Winter Farmers Market. 888 Purchase St, New Bedford, MA 02740. Thursdays 3:00 PM-6:30 PM. Market is open from November to May. Indoor Market on the first floor of the Times Square Building. Street and garage parking available. www.facebook.com/newbedfordfarmersmarket/

Orleans Farmers Market. Main St & Old Colony Way-21 Old Colony Way, Orleans, MA 02653. Saturday, 8:00 AM - Noon. Market is open from May to November. WIC & Senior Coupons Accepted. EBT-SNAP Accepted. Products from Barnstable County exclusively. Vendors: Cape Cod Organic Farm. http://www.orleansfarmersmarket.com/

Osterville Farmers Market. 155 West Bay Road-Osterville Historical Museum, OSTERVILLE, MA 02655. Friday, 9:00 AM - 1:00 PM. Market is open from June to September. WIC & Senior Coupons Accepted. EBT-SNAP accepted with select vendors only. Vendors: Allen Farms,

Cape Cod Organic Farm, Valcourt Sugar Shack, etc.
http://www.ostervillefarmersmarket.org/

Pawtucket Wintertime Farmers Market. Hope Artiste
Village, 1005 Main St, Pawtucket, RI. Saturdays 9:00 AM-
1:00 PM. Market is open from November to April.
Vendors: RI Mushroom co, Allen Farms, Aquidneck Farms,
Freedom Food Farm, Bomster Scallops, Langwater Farm,
Cluck and Trowel, DaSilva Farm, Four town farm, skydog
farm (hydroponic no pesticides), Apponagansett Farm,
Matunuck Oyster Farm, etc.
http://www.farmfreshri.org/2018-pawtucket-wintertime-
farmers-market-vendors/

Plymouth Farmers Market. Plimoth Plantation (grassy
field off River Street), 137 Warren Avenue, Plymouth, MA
02360. Thursday, 2:30 PM- 6:30 PM. Market is open from
May to November. Vendors: Skinny Dip Farm, Plato's
Harvest, Web of Life Organic Farm, Colchester
Neighborhood Farm, Brown Boar Farm, Copicut Farms,
Dufort Farms, Hillside Mushrooms, etc.
PlymouthFarmersMarket.org

Plymouth Winter Farmers Market, Plimouth Plantation,
137 Warren Avenue, Plymouth, MA 02360. Thursdays,
2:30 PM – 6:30 PM. Second Thursday of the month.
Market is open from November to May. SNAP/EBT
accepted.
http://www.plymouthfarmersmarket.org/market-vendors-
indoors-2017/

Plymouth Redbrook Farmers Market. 1 Greenside Way North, Plymouth, MA 02360. GPS address is 237 Wareham Road, Plymouth, MA 02360. Wednesday 3:00 PM – 6:30 PM. Market is open from July to October. https://www.facebook.com/redbrookfarmersmarket/

Provincetown Farmers Market. Commercial St & Ryder St- next to Provincetown Town Hall, Provincetown, MA 02657. Saturday, 9:00 AM - 3:00 PM. Market is open from May to November. WIC & Senior Coupons Accepted. EBT-SNAP Accepted. Vendors: Allen Farms, Silverbrook Farms. https://www.facebook.com/Proviencetownfarmersmarket/

Quincy Farmers Market. Pageant Field at 1 Merrymount Pkwy, Quincy, MA. Friday 11:30 AM – 5:00 PM. Market is open from June to November. Vendors: Ackerman Maple Syrup of VT, Westport Rivers, etc. www.QuincyFarmersMarket.com

Randolph Farmers Market. Powers Farm, 592 North Main Street, Randolph, MA 02368. Wednesday, 3:00 PM - 7:00 PM. Market is open from June to September. WIC & Senior Coupons Accepted. EBT-SNAP accepted. Vendors: Fairmount fruit farm of Franklin [Not organic but use organic or limited pesticides], Freitas Farm, Lane Gardens, and Earthwright Farm. http://mainstreetrandolph.weebly.com/ https://www.facebook.com/Main-Street-Farmers-Market-872816759399636/

Rockland Farmers Market. Plaza in front of Town Hall, 242 Union St., Rockland, MA 02370. Friday 3:00 PM – 6:00 PM. Market is open from June to September. Vendors: Freitas. https://www.facebook.com/farmersmarket02370/

Sandwich Farmers Market. Village Green, 6 Coast Guard Rd., Sandwich, MA 02563. Tuesday, 9:00 AM - 1:00 PM. Market is open from June to October. WIC & Senior Coupons, EBT-SNAP accepted by select vendors only. Vendors: JH Beaulieu Farm, etc. http://www.sandwichfarmersmarket.com/

Scituate Farmers Market. Scituate Harbor, St. Mary's Church parking lot, 1 Kent Street, Scituate, MA. Wednesday, 3:00 PM – 7:00 PM. Market is open from June to October. Vendors: Holly Hill Farms, DaSilva, Brown Boar Farm, Hillside Mushrooms, Overnight Oats [organic oats], E.L. Silvia Farms. www.ScituateFarmersMarket.com

Scituate South Shore Winter Farmers and Artisans Market. St. Luke's Church, 465 First Parish Road, Scituate, MA 02066. Saturday 8:30 AM - 1:00 PM. First and last Saturday of the month. Market is open from January to April. Vendors: DaSilva Farms, Holly Hill Farm, Brown Boar Farm, Foxboro Cheese, https://southshorewinterfarmersandartisansmarket.com/

Sharon Farmers Market. Crescent Ridge Dairy, 407 Bay Road, Sharon, MA. Saturdays 10:00 AM -2:00 PM. Market is open from June to October. Vendors: Da Silva, Wards Berry, etc.www.crescentridgefarmersmarket.com /index.html#vendors

Somerset Open Air Farmers Market. New Hill and Somerset Avenue, Somerset, MA. Saturday (every other) 10:00 AM -2:00 PM. Market is open from June to October. Check their website or Facebook page for latest news, dates, and events. https://www.facebook.com/somersetopenairmarket/

Stoughton Farmers Market. 445 Central Street, Stoughton, MA 02072 [Stoughton Old Colony YMCA]. Monday, 5:00 PM - 7:00 PM. Market is open from June to December. Vendors: Lane Gardens, etc. Website is not working. https://www.facebook.com/StoughtonFarmersMarket/

Swansea Farmers Market. Stoney Creek Farm, 1210 Wilbur Avenue, Swansea MA. Sunday, 10:00 AM -2:00 PM. Market is open from June to October. https://stonycreek-farm.org/swansea-farmers-market-1

Taunton Silver City Farmers Market. Hopewell Park, Hopewell Street, Taunton, MA. Thursday, 3:00 PM to 6:00 PM. Market is open from July to October. https://www.facebook.com/silvercitymarket/ www.massinmotiontaunton.org/the-silver-city-farmers-market.html

Taunton Church Green Farmers Market. First Parish Church, 76 Church Green, Taunton, MA 02780. Sunday, 9:00 AM - 1:00 PM. Market is open from June to October. WIC & Senior Coupons Accepted, EBT-SNAP Accepted. Vendors: Freitas Farm, Green Leaf Gardens, Heart Beets Farm, Breezy Knoll Farm, Coutinho Farm, Lafleurs Wildflower Honey, etc. www.firstparishtaunton.org/church-green-farmers-market.html

Truro Farmers Market. Veteran's Field, 7 Truro Center Road, Truro, MA 02666. Monday, 8:00 AM - Noon. Market is open from June to August. WIC & Senior Coupons, EBT-SNAP accepted. Vendors: Barnstable County grown only. http://www.sustainablecape.org/programs/truro-farmers-market/

Wellfleet Farmers Market. In the Grove at the Congregational Church, 200 Main Street, Wellfleet, MA 02667. Wednesday, 8:00 AM - noon. Market is open from May to October. WIC & Senior Coupons, SNAP accepted. Vendors: Cape Cod Organic Farm, Fleet Town Organics, Wellfleet sea salt co. www.wellfleetfarmersmarket.com/

Weymouth Union Point Farmers Market. The Hangout, 209 Houghton Road, South Weymouth, MA 02190. Sunday, 10:00 AM - 1:00 PM. Market is open from June to October. Vendors: DaSilva Farms, Foxboro Cheese Co., Freitas, Lanni Orchards, Lipinski's Farm, Martha's Vineyard Mushrooms, Red's Best seafood. https://www.weymouth.ma.us/farmers-market OR https://www.facebook.com/weymouthfarmersmarket/

Weymouth Winter Farmers Market. Maria Weston Chapman Middle School cafeteria, 1051 Commercial Street, Weymouth MA 02189. Saturday, 10:00 AM – 1:00 PM. Market is open from January to April. SNAP/EBT accepted.

Yarmouth South /Bass River Farmers Market. 311 Old Main St., South Yarmouth, MA 02664. Thursday and Saturday, 9:00 AM - 1:30 PM. Market is open from June to September. WIC & Senior Coupons, EBT-SNAP accepted with select vendors only. Vendors: Oakdale Farms, Lane Gardens, etc. http://www.bassriverfarmersmarket.org/

FARMERS MARKET MAP

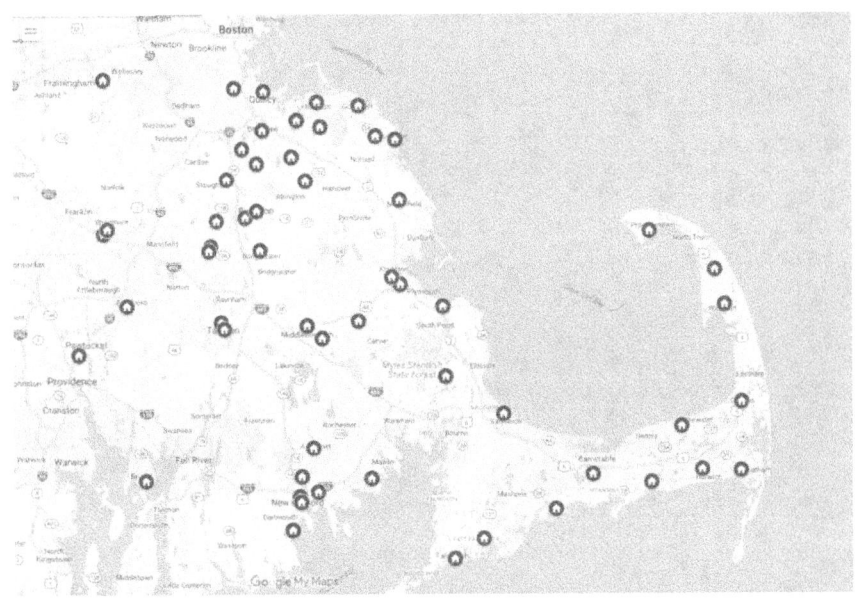

FARMERS MARKET CALENDAR

The following calendar was created in 2018 based on information gathered from multiple sources including the *MassGrown Map*. It includes most markets in and around the South Shore area. This calendar is for reference only. Farmers markets pop up and change locations often. Please call or check websites for the most up-to-date information as days, dates, locations, and times change often.

JANUARY

Look for eggs, cheese, honey, maple syrup, apples, Shitake mushrooms, potatoes, clams, oysters, bay scallops-all in season or available this month and throughout the year.

THURSDAY
New Bedford Winter 3-6:30
Plimoth Plantation WINTER 2:30-6:30 (second Thursday)

SATURDAY
Easton Winter 10-2
Easton @ Simpson Spring 10-2 (year-round)
Falmouth Winter 10-3
Hingham Winter 10-1 (second and fourth Saturday-starts this month)
Marshfield Winter 10-2 (third Saturday)
Mount Hope RI 9-12:30 (year-round)
Natick 9-1 (year-round)
Pawtucket Wintertime 9-1
South Shore Winter Scituate 8:30-1 (First and last Saturday -starts this month)
Weymouth Winter 10-1 (starts this month)

FEBRUARY

Look for eggs, cheese, honey, maple syrup, apples, Shitake mushrooms, potatoes, clams, oysters, bay scallops-all in season or available this month.

TUESDAY
Kingston STONECROFT 3-6 (last Tuesday)

THURSDAY
New Bedford Winter 3-6:30
Plimoth Plantation WINTER 2:30-6:30 (second Thursday)

SATURDAY
Easton Winter 10-2
Easton @ Simpson Spring 10-2 (year-round)
Falmouth Winter 10-3
Hingham Winter 10-1 (second and fourth Saturday)
Marshfield Winter 10-2 (third Saturday)
Mount Hope RI 9-12:30 (year-round)
Natick 9-1 (year-round)
Pawtucket Wintertime 9-1
South Shore Winter Scituate 8:30-1(First and last Saturday)
Weymouth Winter 10-1

MARCH

Look for eggs, cheese, honey, maple syrup, apples, Shitake mushrooms, potatoes, clams, oysters, bay scallops-all in season or available this month.

TUESDAY
Kingston STONECROFT 3-6 (last Tuesday)

THURSDAY
New Bedford Winter 3-6:30
Plimoth Plantation WINTER 2:30-6:30 (second Thursday)

SATURDAY
Easton Winter 10-2
Easton @ Simpson Spring 10-2 (year-round)
Falmouth Winter 10-3
Hingham Winter 10-1 (second and fourth Saturday-ends this month)
Marshfield Winter 10-2 (third Saturday)
Mount Hope RI 9-12:30 (year-round)
Natick 9-1 (year-round)
Pawtucket Wintertime 9-1
South Shore Winter Scituate 8:30-1 (First and last Saturday)
Weymouth Winter 10-1

APRIL

Look for eggs, cheese, honey, maple syrup, apples, Shitake mushrooms, potatoes, clams, oysters, bay scallops-all in season or available this month.

TUESDAY
Kingston STONECROFT 3-6 (last Tuesday)

THURSDAY
New Bedford Winter 3-6:30
Plimoth Plantation WINTER 2:30-6:30 (second Thursday)

SATURDAY
Easton Winter 10-2
Easton @ Simpson Spring 10-2 (year-round)
Falmouth Winter 10-3 (ends this month)
Hingham Winter 10-1 (second and last Saturday)
Marshfield Winter 10-2 (third Saturday)
Mount Hope RI 9-12:30 (year-round)
Natick 9-1 (year-round)
Pawtucket Wintertime 9-1 (ends this month)
South Shore Winter Scituate 8:30-1 (First and last Saturday- ends this month)
Weymouth Winter 10-1 (ends this month)

MAY

Look for asparagus, Edible Flowers, Fiddleheads (this month only), horseradish, lettuce, scallions and spinach- all in season or available this month.

TUESDAY
Chatham 3-6 (starts this month)
Kingston STONECROFT 3-6 (last Tuesday- starts this month)

WEDNESDAY
Wellfleet 8-noon (starts this month)

THURSDAY
New Bedford Winter 3-6:30 (ends this month)
Plimoth Plantation WINTER2:30-6:30 (second Thursday-ends this month)
Plimoth Plantation SUMMER 2:30-6:30 (starts this month)
Falmouth 12-6 (starts this month)

FRIDAY
Hyannis Summer 3-6 (starts this month)

SATURDAY
Easton Winter 10-2 (ends this month)
Easton Summer 10-2 (starts this month)
Easton @ Simpson Spring 10-2 (year-round)
Hingham Summer 10-2 (starts this month)
Marshfield Winter 10-2 (third Saturday-ends this month)
Mount Hope RI 9-12:30 (year-round)
Natick 9-1 (year-round)
Orleans 8-noon (starts this month)
Pawtucket Wintertime 9-1
Provincetown 9-3 (starts this month)

JUNE

Look for strawberries and Cherries , arugula, beets, bok choy, cabbage, cauliflower, cucumbers, Gooseberries , elderberry, lettuce, peas, radishes, scallions and spinach-all in season or available this month.

SUNDAY
Brewster 9-1 (starts this month)
Carver Noon-4 (starts this month)
Fairhaven 11-3 (starts this month)
Kingston Collection Way 10-2 (first Sunday of month-starts this month)
Swansea 10-2 (starts this month)
Taunton Church Green 9-1 (starts this month)
Weymouth Union Point 10-1 (starts this month)

MONDAY
New Bedford Brooklawn Park 2-6 (starts this month)
Stoughton 5p-7pm (starts this month)
Truro 8-noon (starts this month)

TUESDAY
Bridgewater, West 4-7 PM (select dates) (starts this month)
Chatham 3-6
Kingston STONECROFT 3-6 (last Tuesday only)
Mattapoisett 3-6 (starts this month)
Sandwich 9-1(starts this month)

WEDNESDAY
Randolph 3-7 (starts this month)
Scituate 3-7 (starts this month)
Wellfleet 8-noon

THURSDAY
Cohasset 2-6 (starts this month)
Falmouth 12-6
Harwich 3-6 (starts this month)
Milton 1-6 (starts this month)
New Bedford Custom House 2-6 (starts this month)
Plimoth Plantation 2:30-6:30
Yarmouth, South 9-1:30 (starts this month)

82

FRIDAY
Brockton City Hall 10-2
Dartmouth 1-6 (starts this month)
Hyannis 3-6
Marshfield 2-6 (starts this month)
Osterville 9-1 (starts this month)
Quincy 11:30-5 (starts this month)
Rockland Town Hall 3-6 (starts this month)

SATURDAY
Acushnet 8-1:30 (starts this month)
Andover10-2 (starts this month)
Attleboro 9-1 (starts this month)
Braintree 9-1 (starts this month)
Brewster 9-1(starts this month)
Easton Summer 10-2
Easton @ Simpson Spring 10-2 (year-round)
Hingham Summer 10-2
Holbrook 9-2 (starts this month)
Middleboro 10-2 (starts this month)
Middleborough 9:30-1 (starts this month)
Mount Hope RI 9-12:30 (year-round)
Natick 9-1 (year-round)
New Bedford Clasky 10-2 (starts this month)
Orleans 8-noon
Provincetown 9-3
Sharon 10-2 (starts this month)
Somerset 10-2 (every other Saturday-starts this month)
Yarmouth, South 9-1:30 (starts this month)

JULY

Look for apples, blueberries, peaches (late July),raspberries, arugula, green beans, beets, bok choy, broccoli, cabbage, carrots, cauliflower, chard, corn on the cob, cucumbers, eggplant, garlic, lettuce, onions, peas, peppers, radishes, scallions, spinach and zucchini -all in season or available this month.

SUNDAY
Brewster 9-1
Carver Noon-4
Fairhaven 11-3
Kingston Collection Way 10-2 (first Sunday only)
Taunton Church Green 9-1
Swansea 10-2
Weymouth Union Point 10-1

MONDAY
New Bedford Brooklawn Park 2-6
Stoughton 5p-7pm
Truro 8-noon

TUESDAY
Bridgewater, West 4-7 PM
Chatham 3-6
Kingston STONECROFT 3-6 (last Tuesday)
Mattapoisett 3-6
Sandwich 9-1

WEDNESDAY
Plymouth Redbrook 3-6 (starts this month)
Randolph 3-7
Scituate 3-7
Wellfleet 8-noon

THURSDAY
Cohasset 2-6
Falmouth 12-6
Harwich 3-6
Milton 1-6
New Bedford 2-6
Plimoth Plantation 2:30-6:30
Taunton 3-6 (starts this month)
Yarmouth, South 9-1:30

FRIDAY
Brockton City Hall 10-2 (starts this month)
Dartmouth 1-6
Hyannis 3-6
Marshfield 2-6
Osterville 9-1
Quincy 11:30-5
Rockland Town Hall 3-6

SATURDAY
Acushnet 8-1:30
Andover10-2
Attleboro 9-1
Braintree 9-1
Brewster 9-1
Brockton Fairgrounds 9-noon (starts this month)
Easton 10-2
Easton @ Simpson Spring 10-2 (year-round)
Hingham 10-2
Holbrook 9-2
Middleboro 10-2
Middleborough 9:30-1
Mount Hope RI 9-12:30 (year-round)
Natick 9-1 (year-round)
New Bedford Clasky 10-2
Orleans 8-noon
Provincetown 9-3
Sharon 10-2
Somerset 10-2 (every other Saturday)
Yarmouth, South 9-1:30

AUGUST

Look for apples, arugula, blueberries, green beans, beets, bok choy, broccoli, cabbage, Cantaloupe (this month only), carrots, cauliflower, celery, chard, corn on the cob, cucumbers, eggplant, figs, garlic, grapes, green beans, lettuce, nectarines, onions, peas, peaches , peppers, plums, radishes, raspberries, scallions, spinach, watermelon and zucchini -all in season or available this month.

SUNDAY
Brewster 9-1
Carver Noon-4
Fairhaven 11-3
Kingston Collection Way 10-2 (first Sunday only)
Swansea 10-2
Taunton Church Green 9-1
Weymouth Union Point 10-1

MONDAY
New Bedford Brooklawn Park 2-6
Stoughton 5p-7pm
Truro 8-noon (ends this month)

TUESDAY
Bridgewater, West 4-7 PM (ends this month)
Chatham 3-6
Kingston STONECROFT 3-6 (last Tuesday)
Mattapoisett 3-6
Sandwich 9-1

WEDNESDAY
Plymouth Redbrook 3-6
Randolph 3-7
Scituate 3-7
Wellfleet 8-noon

THURSDAY
Cohasset 2-6
Falmouth 12-6
Harwich 3-6
Milton 1-6
New Bedford 2-6
Plimoth Plantation 2:30-6:30
Taunton 3-6
Yarmouth, South 9-1:30

FRIDAY
Brockton City Hall 10-2
Dartmouth 1-6
Hyannis 3-6
Marshfield 2-6
Osterville 9-1
Quincy 11:30-5
Rockland Town Hall 3-6

SATURDAY
Acushnet 8-1:30
Andover10-2
Attleboro 9-1
Braintree 9-1
Brewster 9-1
Brockton Fairgrounds 9-12
Easton 10-2
Easton @ Simpson Spring 10-2 (year-round)
Hingham 10-2
Holbrook 9-2
Middleboro 10-2
Middleborough 9:30-1
Mount Hope RI 9-12:30 (year-round)
Natick 9-1 (year-round)
New Bedford Clasky 10-2
Orleans 8-noon
Provincetown 9-3
Sharon 10-2
Somerset 10-2 (every other Saturday)
Yarmouth, South 9-1:30

SEPTEMBER

Look for apples, arugula, blueberries, beets, bok choy, broccoli, cabbage, carrots, cauliflower, celery, corn on the cob, cranberries, cucumbers, eggplant, fennel, ginger, grapes, green beans, lettuce, Lingonberries, nectarines, onions, peas, peaches , pear-Asian, peppers, plums, radishes, raspberries, spinach, watermelon and zucchini -all in season or available this month.

SUNDAY
Brewster 9-1(ends this month)
Carver Noon-4
Fairhaven 11-3
Kingston Collection Way 10-2 (first Sunday only)
Swansea 10-2
Taunton Church Green 9-1
Weymouth Union Point 10-1

MONDAY
New Bedford Brooklawn Park 2-6
Stoughton 5p-7pm

TUESDAY
Chatham 3-6
Kingston STONECROFT 3-6 (last Tuesday of the month only)
Mattapoisett 3-6
Sandwich 9-1

WEDNESDAY
Plymouth Redbrook 3-6
Randolph 3-7 (ends this month)
Scituate 3-7
Wellfleet 8-noon

THURSDAY
Cohasset 2-6
Falmouth 12-6
Harwich 3-6
Milton 1-6
New Bedford Custom House 2-6
Plimoth Plantation 2:30-6:30
Taunton 3-6
Yarmouth, South 9-1:30 (ends this month)

FRIDAY
Brockton City Hall 10-2
Dartmouth 1-6
Hyannis Summer Market 3-6 (ends this month)
Marshfield 2-6
Osterville 9-1 (ends this month)
Quincy 11:30-5
Rockland Town Hall 3-6 (ends this month)

SATURDAY
Acushnet 8-1:30 (ends this month)
Andover10-2
Attleboro 9-1
Braintree 9-1
Brewster 9-1 (ends this month)
Brockton Fairgrounds 9-12
Easton 10-2
Easton @ Simpson Spring 10-2 (year-round)
Hingham 10-2
Holbrook 9-2
Middleboro 10-2
Middleborough 9:30-1
Mount Hope RI 9-12:30 (year-round)
Natick 9-1 (year-round)
New Bedford Clasky 10-2
Orleans 8-noon
Provincetown 9-3
Sharon 10-2
Somerset 10-2 (every other Saturday)
Yarmouth, South 9-1:30 (ends this month)

OCTOBER

Look for apples, arugula, beets, bok choy, broccoli, cabbage, carrots, cauliflower, celery, corn on the cob, cranberries, cucumbers, eggplant, fennel, ginger, grapes, green beans, lettuce, Lingonberries, nectarines, onions, peas, pear-Asian, peppers, radishes, raspberries, spinach, tomatillos, watermelon and zucchini -all in season or available this month.

SUNDAY
Carver Noon-4 (ends this month)
Fairhaven 11-3 (ends this month)
Kingston Collection Way 10-2 (first Sunday only-ends this month)
Swansea 10-2 (ends this month)
Taunton Church Green 9-1 (ends this month)
Weymouth Union Point 10-1 (ends this month)

MONDAY
New Bedford Brooklawn Park 2-6 (ends this month)
Stoughton 5p-7pm

TUESDAY
Chatham 3-6 (ends this month)
Kingston STONECROFT 3-6 (last Tuesday only- ends this month)
Mattapoisett 3-6 (ends this month)
Sandwich 9-1 (ends this month)

WEDNESDAY
Plymouth Redbrook 3-6 (ends this month)
Scituate 3-7 (ends this month)
Wellfleet 8-noon (ends this month)

THURSDAY

Cohasset 2-6 (ends this month)
Falmouth Summer 12-6 (ends this month)
Harwich 3-6 (ends this month)
New Bedford Custom House 2-6 (ends this month)
Milton 1-6 (ends this month)
Plimoth Plantation 2:30-6:30
Taunton 3-6 (ends this month)

FRIDAY

Brockton City Hall 10-2 (ends this month)
Dartmouth 1-6 (ends this month)
Marshfield 2-6 (ends this month)
Quincy 11:30-5

SATURDAY

Andover10-2 (ends this month)
Attleboro 9-1 (ends this month)
Braintree 9-1 (ends this month)
Brockton Fairgrounds 9-12 (ends this month)
Easton Summer 10-2 (ends this month)
Easton @ Simpson Spring 10-2 (year-round)
Hingham 10-2
Holbrook 9-2 (ends this month)
Middleboro 10-2 (ends this month)
Middleborough 9:30-1 (ends this month)
Mount Hope RI 9-12:30 (year-round)
Natick 9-1 (year-round)
New Bedford Clasky 10-2 (ends this month)
Orleans 8-noon
Provincetown 9-3
Sharon 10-2 (ends this month)
Somerset 10-2 (every other Saturday-ends this month)
Yarmouth, South 9-1:30

NOVEMBER

Look for apples, cranberries, broccoli, cabbage, carrots, garlic, onions, pear-Asian and pumpkins-all in season or available this month.

MONDAY
Stoughton 5p-7pm

TUESDAY
Kingston STONECROFT 3-6 (last Tuesday of month)

THURSDAY
New Bedford Winter 3-6:30 (starts this month)
Plimoth Plantation SUMMER 2:30-6:30 (ends this month)
Plimoth Plantation WINTER 2:30-6:30 (second Thursday of month- starts this month)

FRIDAY
Quincy 11:30-5 (ends this month)

SATURDAY
Easton Winter 10-2 (starts this month)
Easton @ Simpson Spring 10-2 (year-round)
Falmouth Winter 10-3 (starts this month)
Hingham Summer 10-2 (ends this month)
Hyannis Winter 11-4 (starts this month)
Marshfield Winter 10-2 (third Saturday-starts this month)
Mount Hope RI 9-12:30 (year-round)
Natick 9-1 (year-round)
Orleans 8-noon (ends this month)
Pawtucket Wintertime 9-1(starts this month)
Provincetown 9-3 (ends this month)

DECEMBER

Look for apples, cranberries, beets, broccoli, cabbage, carrots, garlic, parsnips, pear-Asian and potatoes-all in season or available this month.

MONDAY
Stoughton 5p-7PM (ends this month)

TUESDAY
Kingston STONECROFT 3-6 (last Tuesday)

THURSDAY
New Bedford Winter 3-6:30
Plimoth Plantation WINTER 2:30-6:30 (second Thursday of month)

SATURDAY
Easton Winter 10-2
Easton @ Simpson Spring 10-2 (year-round)
Falmouth Winter 10-3
Hyannis Winter 11-4 (ends this month)
Mount Hope RI 9-12:30 (year-round)
Natick 9-1 (year-round)
Marshfield Winter 10-2 (third Saturday)
Northampton Winter 9-2
Pawtucket Wintertime 9-1

PRODUCE AVAILABILITY CALENDAR

Produce ripens or is available in New England around the same time every year. But, several factors affect the exact date and availability of crops. Factors include too much rain, not enough sun, not enough rain, severe storms that damage crops, and pest infestation, to name a few. The following chart shows a rough range of crop availability based on past years. Always call ahead, review Facebook or the webpage of a farm before you visit in order to know what products are available that day. Sometimes a crop is ready but due to high demand or low yield they have run out for the day thus another reason to call ahead.

The following data was collected from various sources including; Farm Fresh RI[xiv], Massachusetts Seasonal Food Guide[xv], and the Massachusetts Department of Agricultural Resources.[xvi]

JANUARY

Beets

Broccoli

Brussel Sprouts

Cabbage

Collards

Kale

Leeks

Microgreens

Mushrooms; Black Trumpet,
Chanterelle, Hedgehog,
White Truffle

Shallots

Sprouts

FEBRUARY

Brussel Sprouts

Cabbage

Collards

Kale

Leeks

Microgreens

Mushrooms; Black Trumpet,
Chanterelle, Hedgehog,
White Truffle

Sprouts

MARCH

Brussel Sprouts

Chives

Collards

Horseradish

Kale

Microgreens

Mint

Morels

Mushrooms; Black Trumpet,
Chanterelle, Hedgehog,
White Truffle

Nettles

Ramps

Sprouts

APRIL

Asparagus

Chives

Collards

Edible Flowers

Fiddleheads

Horseradish

Kale

Lettuce

Microgreens

Mint

Morels

Mushrooms; Morel

Nettles

Parsnips

Ramps

Sprouts

Watercress

MAY

Arugula

Asparagus

Bok Choi

Chives

Collards

Dandelion

Edible Flowers

Fiddleheads

Garlic fresh, uncured

Garlic Scapes

Horseradish

Kale

Lambsquarters

Leeks

Lettuce

Microgreens

Mint

Morels

Mushrooms; Morel, Porcini, Chanterelle

Nettles

Parsnips

Radishes (edible greens)

Ramps

Rhubarb

Sprouts

Strawberries

Watercress

JUNE

Arugula

Asparagus

Beets

Blueberries

Bok Choi

Broccoli

Cabbage

Cauliflower

Cherries

Chives

Dandelion

Edible Flowers

Elderberry

Endive

Escarole

Fava beans

Fennel

Garlic fresh, uncured

Garlic Scapes

Gooseberries

Green beans

Horseradish

Kale

Kohlrabi

Lambsquarters

Leeks

Lettuce

Microgreens

Mint

Mushrooms; Morel, Porcini,
Chanterelle

Peas, snap

Purslane

Radishes (edible greens)

Ramps

Rhubarb

Shallots

Shell Beans

Snap Peas

Snow Peas

Sorrel

Spinach

Sprouts

Strawberries

Watercress

JULY

Artichokes

Arugula

Beets

Blueberries

Bok Choi

Broccoli

Cabbage

Carrots

Cauliflower

Celery

Chili peppers

Chives

Collards

Corn

Cucumbers

Currants

Dandelion

Edible Flowers

Eggplant

Elderberry

Elderflower

Fava beans

Fennel

Garlic fresh, uncured

Garlic Scapes

Gooseberries

Green beans

Horseradish

Jostaberries

Kale

Kohlrabi

Lambsquarters

Leeks

Lettuce

Microgreens

Mint

Mushrooms; Lobster, Chanterelle

Okra

Onions, uncured or with greens

Peaches

Peas, snap

Peppers

Purslane

Radishes (edible greens)

Raspberries

Rhubarb

Shallots

Shell Beans

Snap Peas

Snow Peas

Sorrel

Spinach

Sprouts

Summer Squash

Sunchokes

Watercress

Zucchini

AUGUST

Apples

Artichokes

Arugula

Beets

Blueberries

Bok Choi

Broccoli

Brussel Sprouts

Cabbage

Carrots

Cauliflower

Celery

Celery Root aka Celeriac

Chili peppers

Chives

Collards

Corn

Cucumbers

Currants

Dandelion

Edamame

Edible Flowers

Eggplant

Fava beans

Fennel

Figs

Garlic fresh, uncured

Ginger

Gooseberries

Grapes

Green beans

Horseradish

Jostaberries

Kale

Kohlrabi

Lambsquarters

Leeks

Lettuce

Lima Beans

Melons

Microgreens

Mint

Mushrooms, Lobster, Chanterelle

Nectarines

Okra

Onions, uncured or with greens

Peaches

Peas, snap

Peppers

Plums

Purslane

Radishes (edible greens)

Raspberries

Rhubarb

Rutabaga

Shell Beans

Snap Peas

Snow Peas

Sorrel

Spinach

Sprouts

Strawberries

Summer Squash

Sweet potatoes

Turnips

Watermelon

Zucchini

SEPTEMBER

Apples

Arugula

Beets

Blueberries

Bok Choi

Broccoli

Brussel Sprouts

Cabbage

Carrots

Cauliflower

Celery

Celery Root aka Celeriac

Chili peppers

Chives

Collards

Corn

Cranberries

Cucumbers

Edamame

Edible Flowers

Eggplant

Endive

Escarole

Fava beans

Fennel

Ginger

Grapes

Green beans

Horseradish

Kale

Kohlrabi

Lambsquarters

Leeks

Lettuce

Lima Beans

Lingonberries

Microgreens

Mushrooms; Lobster, Chanterelle, Matsutake

Nectarines

Okra

Onions, uncured or with greens

Peaches

Pear, Asian

Peas, snap

Peppers

Plums

potatoes

pumpkin

Purslane

Quince

Radicchio

Radishes (edible greens)

Raspberries

Rutabaga

Shell Beans

Snap Peas

Snow Peas

Sorrel

Spinach

Sprouts

Strawberries

Summer Squash

Sweet potatoes

Tomatillos

Tomatoes

Turnips

Watermelon

Winter Squash

Zucchini

OCTOBER

Apples

Arugula

Beets

Bok Choi

Broccoli

Brussel Sprouts

Cabbage

Carrots

Cauliflower

Celery

Chili peppers

Collards

Corn

Cranberries

Cucumbers

Edamame

Eggplant

Endive

Escarole

Fennel

Ginger

Green beans

Horseradish

Kale

Kohlrabi

Leeks

Lettuce

Lima Beans

Lingonberries

Microgreens

Mushrooms; Matsutake

Okra

Onions, uncured or with greens

Parsnips

Pear, Asian

Peas, snap

Peppers

potatoes

pumpkin

Purslane

Quince

Radicchio

Rutabaga

Snap Peas

Snow Peas

Sorrel

Spinach

Sprouts

Tomatillos

Tomatoes

Turnips

Watermelon

Winter Squash

NOVEMBER

Arugula

Beets

Bok Choi

Broccoli

Brussel Sprouts

Cabbage

Carrots

Cauliflower

Celery

Collards

Cranberries

Endive

Escarole

Fennel

Green beans

Horseradish

Kale

Leeks

Lettuce

Microgreens

Mushrooms; Matsutake, White Truffle

Onions, uncured or with greens

Parsnips

Peppers

Potatoes

pumpkin

Quince

Rutabaga   Sprouts

Sprouts

DECEMBER

Beets

Broccoli

Brussel Sprouts

Cabbage

Carrots

Cauliflower

Collards

Cranberries

Kale

Leeks

Microgreens

Mushrooms; Black Trumpet,
Chanterelle, Hedgehog,
White Truffle

Parsnips

Potatoes

Shallots

SUPERMARKET CHEAT SHEET

When shopping at your local grocery store bring along this cheat sheet to remember what NOT to buy. Read the labels of packaged foods. And avoid the following conventionally grown produce.

AVOID	AVOID CONVENTIONAL
Canola	Alfalfa
Canola oil	Apples
Corn oil	Beans, Green
Corn starch	Beets (Sugar)
Corn Syrup	Celery
Cottonseed oil	Cherries
Granulated sugar	Corn
High-fructose corn syrup	Grapes
Soy lecithin	Kale
Soybean oil	Lettuce
	Nectarines
	Papaya
	Peaches
	Pears
	Peppers, Sweet bell
	Potatoes
	Soybean
	Spinach
	Squash
	Strawberries
	Tomatoes

GLOSSARY

The following glossary of terms were copied from various sources including; the USDA.gov, ucanr.edu, sierraclub.org, seacoastharvest.org.

Aquaponics: a method of producing food that combines raising aquatic animals (such as fish or shrimp) and plants. The waste from the animals is used as fertilizer for the plants.

Biodynamic: a method of farming developed by Rudolf Steiner, an Austrian scientist and philosopher. This approach regards a farm as a self-contained, living organism and emphasizes the vitality of soil maintenance and composting. Biodynamic growers work to balance and consider both the physical and non-physical aspects and cycles of a farm in their production.

Biological Control/Bio-control: "Biological control is, generally, human's use of a specially chosen living organism to control a particular pest. This chosen organism might be a predator, parasite, or disease which will attack the harmful insect. It is a form of manipulating nature to increase a desired effect. A complete Biological Control program may range from choosing a pesticide which will be least harmful to beneficial insects, to raising and releasing one insect to have it attack another, almost like a 'living insecticide.'" [David Orr, Steve Bambara, and James Baker, *Biological Pest Control: An Introduction* (Center for IPM, North Carolina State University, 1997).

Cage Free: Cage Free describes poultry that was not raised in cages. However, it is also important to know what the birds were fed and if they were allowed access to pasture and fresh air.

Certified Farmers' Market (CFM): locations where farmers and ranchers are allowed to sell directly to customers, exempt from USDA packaging, sizing, and labeling regulations. These locations must be certified by the County Agricultural Commissioner. Many CFMs have technically separate, but adjacent markets where prepared food, bread and other complimentary items may be sold. Farmers may also sell direct to consumers at farm stands.

Certified Naturally Grown: The farm is certified by the nonprofit Certified Naturally Grown, an alternative to the USDA's National Organic Program (NOP). The standards and growing requirements are no less strict than the NOP rules.

Community Supported Agriculture (CSA): a farm that is funded by a group of community members. Members pay an annual or quarterly fee in exchange for a weekly assortment of farm fresh produce or other farm products. CSA helps local farmers increase cash flow and diversifies risk over multiple crops.

Conventional Agriculture: the modern form of industrialized agriculture which emphasizes maximum productivity and profitability, practiced on the majority of US farms. Conventional agriculture is characterized by mechanization, monocultures, and the use of synthetic fertilizers and pesticides. Conventional agriculture may also use genetically modified organisms. This form of industrialized agriculture has become "conventional" only within the last 60 years or so.

Crop rotation: planting different crops on the land in successive years. Modern industrial agriculture involves rotating between corn and soybeans in successive years. More sustainable farming practices would include several more crops besides corn and soybeans, such as hay, oats and rye.

Farmers market: a retail market where farmers sell their produce, meat and eggs directly to the consumers. Some farmers markets sell prepared foods and wines.

Free- Range: livestock or poultry that is permitted to forage in large area of open land rather than confined to a feedlot. According to the USDA "free range" must have access to the outdoors, but the amount or quality is not regulated. Animals are given daily access to the outdoors, but are not raised primarily on pasture.

Grass-fed (100%): Animals only eat grasses from start to finish.

Grass-fed with Grain Supplement: Animals are raised on pasture, and a controlled amount of grain is eventually introduced into their diet.

Genetically Modified Organism (GMO): an organism that has been altered genetically, typically through the transfer of DNA from another organism. Alterations result in the expression of new characteristics not naturally belonging to that organism. Genetic modification is currently allowed in conventional agriculture in the United States. (also Genetic Engineering)

Grass Fed: a USDA standard requiring that an animal's only feed source be grass or forage, except for milk consumed prior to weaning. Animals are required to have continuous access to pasture during the growing season. Grass-fed animals may not be fed grain or grain by-products at any time during their lifetime.

Heirloom v. Hybrid v. GMO: Heirloom vegetables are vegetables whose seeds have been saved for generations and passed down. By contrast, seeds from hybrid plants are not true to type and so are not good for saving. This requires that the grower purchase new seeds every year. Hybrids have been bred for specific qualities but have not been genetically modified. GMO plants have been genetically engineered. This can be done by combining DNA of different plant varieties or by introducing genes from other species, such as fish.

Heritage Breeds: The farm raises rare and endangered breeds of livestock to reintroduce genetic diversity and prevent extinction.

Integrated Pest Management aka IPM: The farm uses a pest-management strategy that includes a combination of biological, cultural, and chemical tools to reduce crop damage from insects, diseases and weeds. Pesticides are used minimally and judiciously as only one part of the pest management strategy. See also Biological Control.

Low-spray (fruit): The farm uses a reduced synthetic pesticide spray program relative to the region's conventional spray practices.

No-till: "The practice of planting new crops amidst cuttings of old crops and not plowing the field in order to slow the release of carbon dioxide and diminish the greenhouse effect. No-till and low-till practices also increase the retention of water and nutrients, allowing earthworms and other organisms to proliferate and keep the soil healthy."

Organic: a USDA standard that requires that crops are raised without the use of most conventional pesticides, petroleum or sewage-based fertilizers, or genetically engineered materials. There is an emphasis on using renewable resources and conservation. Animal products must come from animals that have been fed organic feed, had access to the outdoors, and received neither antibiotics nor growth hormones. Meat products must also be processed in an organic certified facility. The use of the term Organic is regulated by the USDA, and is only permissible by certified producers.

Pasture-Raised: Animals are raised outdoors on pasture in a humane, ecologically sustainable manner, rather than in a feedlot or confined facility.

Sustainable Agriculture: an approach that encompasses a wide variety of methods of farming and ranching with the common goals of providing more farm profits, achieving greater environmental stewardship, and benefiting their families and communities. Some common practices include protecting and improving soil quality, reducing dependence on fuel, synthetic fertilizers and pesticides, and minimizing adverse impacts on wildlife, water quality and other environmental resource.

Transitional: The farm follows organic management practices, but has not yet fulfilled time requirements to be certified organic (land must be free of prohibited materials for a minimum of 3 years to be certified).

USDA CERTIFIED ORGANIC: According to the United States Department of Agriculture's website *USDA.gov*, "USDA certified organic foods are grown and processed according to federal guidelines addressing, among many factors, soil quality, animal raising practices, pest and weed control, and use of additives. Organic producers rely on natural substances and physical, mechanical, or biologically based farming methods to the fullest extent possible. Produce can be called organic if it's certified to have grown on soil that had no prohibited substances applied for three years prior to harvest. Prohibited substances include most synthetic fertilizers and pesticides. In instances when a grower has to use a synthetic substance to achieve a specific purpose, the substance must first be approved according to criteria that examine its effects on human health and the environment... As with all organic foods, none of it is grown or handled using genetically modified organisms, which the organic standards expressly prohibit."

SOURCES

100 mile diet, Eco life; a guide to green living, an overview of the 100-mile diet, by Maryruth Belsey Priebe, http://www.ecolife.com/health-food/eating-local/100-mile-diet.html

Cape Cod Buy Fresh Buy Local, Barnstable, MA, Connects people on Cape Cod with locally grown farm and sea products, through education and information. https://www.buyfreshbuylocalcapecod.org/

Certified Naturally Grown, grassroots certification that builds farms and communities, https://certified.naturallygrown.org

Consumer Reports, Greener Choices, http://greenerchoices.org

Eat Wild, Getting Wild Nutrition from Modern Food, http://www.eatwild.com/

Edible South Shore and South Coast, Shop Local, http://ediblesouthshore.com/

Environmental Working Group (EWG), know your environment. Protect your health. EWG is a non-profit, non-partisan organization dedicated to protecting human health and the environment, https://www.ewg.org

Farm Fresh RI, A hub for local food since 2004, Programs, Farmers Markets, www.farmfreshri.org/programs/farmers-markets/

Farmers Market Coalition, The Farmers Market Coalition is a 501(c)(3) nonprofit dedicated to strengthening farmers markets across the United States so that they can serve as community assets while providing real income opportunities for farmers. https://farmersmarketcoalition.org/

Federation of Massachusetts Farmers Markets, Waltham, MA. FMFM works to improve the health of individuals, strengthen community vitality, and enhance local farm viability through farmers markets. http://illdave.com/web/fmfm/federation/about.htm

Florida Department of Agriculture and Consumer Services, Divisions & Offices, Marketing and development, Consumer Resources, Buy "Fresh from Florida", https://www.freshfromflorida.com/

GMO Answers, GMO Answers was created to do a better job answering your questions — no matter what they are — about GMOs. Current GMO crops, https://gmoanswers.com/current-gmo-crops

Grace Communications Foundation Inc., Seasonal Food Guide, Find what's in season near you, Massachusetts Seasonal Food Guide, https://www.seasonalfoodguide.org/massachusetts/

Homegrown, Farm Aid created homegrown.org to be a place where we connect to the land and to each other. http://www.homegrown.org/

Island Grown Initiative, Martha's Vineyard. We support a resilient & equitable food system on Martha's Vineyard by providing food and agriculture education and developing infrastructure to make a year-round local food system viable. http://www.igimv.org/

Land For Good. Working to ensure the future of farming in New England by putting more farmers more securely on more land. http://landforgood.org/

Living Non-Gmo, a lifestyle site created by the non-gmo project, https://livingnongmo.org/learn/resources/

Local Harvest, Real food, real farmers, real community, https://www.localharvest.org

Local Farm Markets, Southeast Massachusetts, Find a real local farmer's market, roadside stand, or farm stand near you. http://www.localfarmmarkets.org/MAsefarmmarkets.php

Massachusetts Agricultural Fairs Association, Abington, Encourages, promotes and preserves agricultural activities in the commonwealth through its members and their individual programs. http://www.mafa.org/

Massachusetts Aquaculture Association, Eastham, Its purpose is to promote the continued development of shellfish and fish farming, and to improve conditions affecting aquaculture in Massachusetts. https://massaquaculture.wordpress.com/

Massachusetts Association of Roadside Stands and Pick Your Own.

Massachusetts Audubon Society, Lincoln. Serves as a leader and a catalyst for conservation, by acting directly to protect nature, and by stimulating individual and institutional action. https://www.massaudubon.org/

Massachusetts Department of Agricultural Resources, MDAR, The Department's mission is to help keep the Massachusetts' food supply safe and secure, and to work to keep Massachusetts agriculture economically and environmentally sound, https://www.mass.gov/orgs/massachusetts-department-of-agricultural-resources

Massachusetts Department of Environmental Protection, Boston. A state agency that ensures clean air and water, manages toxics safely, coordinates waste recycling, and preserves wetlands and coastal resources. https://www.mass.gov/orgs/massachusetts-department-of-environmental-protection

Massachusetts Farm Bureau Federation, Marlborough. An independent, non-governmental, voluntary organization representing agriculture in the Commonwealth of Massachusetts. http://www.mfbf.net/

Massachusetts Farm Wineries & Growers Association. Encourages consumer awareness of Massachusetts wines and promotes a positive business environment for continued growth and production of Massachusetts grown wines. http://www.masswinery.com/

Massachusetts Lobstermen's Association. Scituate. A member-driven organization that accepts and supports the interdependence of species conservation and the members' collective economic interests. http://lobstermen.com/

Massachusetts Local Food Action Plan. In 2013 the Massachusetts Food Policy Council launched a statewide planning process to address the opportunities and challenges of our State's local food system. The Plan was completed and accepted by the Council in December 2015. https://mafoodsystem.org/plan/

Massachusetts Maple Producers Association, Plainfield. A nonprofit organization dedicated to the preservation and promotion of maple sugaring in Massachusetts. https://www.massmaple.org

Massachusetts Natural Resources Collaborations, MASSNRC, https://massnrc.org

Massachusetts Food System Collaborative. The goals of the Collaborative are to promote, monitor, and facilitate implementation of the 2015 Massachusetts Local Food Action Plan. https://mafoodsystem.org

Massachusetts State Grange. Promotes local agriculture and agricultural education, through local granges and through partnerships with other organizations. http://www.massgrange.org/

Mass Farmers Markets, Waltham, MA, manages the Copley Square market, Central Square market, and Davis Square Market. http://massfarmersmarkets.org/

MassGrown, Massachusetts Grown...and Fresher. It is your gateway to farms, farmers markets, and fun ag-tivities!! We will keep you up to date on seasonal crops and products grown in Massachusetts. https://www.mass.gov/orgs/massachusetts-grownand-fresher

National Organic Program (NOP), a program within the USDA marketing service. Responsible for developing national standards for organic products. https://www.ams.usda.gov

One Green Planet, Welcome to Green Monsters! We're your online guide to making conscious choices that help people, animals and the planet, http://www.onegreenplanet.org

New England Vegetable and Berry Growers Association, Amherst. Supports and promotes the vegetable and berry industry in New England. http://nevbga.org/index.php

New Entry Sustainable Farming Project, Lowell, MA. Provides critical training, career development, and economic opportunity to new farmers. An entrepreneur's guide to farming in Massachusetts. https://nesfp.org/

Northeast Organic Farming Association, NOFA MASS, the Massachusetts chapter of the Northeast Organic Farming Association, NOFA/Mass welcomes everyone who cares about food, where it comes from and how it's grown, https://www.nofamass.org/

Seacoast Harvest, You resource for finding locally grown food in Rockingham, Strafford and York Counties of NH & Maine, Local Food Guide, A project of Seacoast eat local, Farmers Markets, Seafood, Agricultural Glossary, Harvest Calendar, Printable Guide, seacoastharvest.org

Southeastern Massachusetts Agricultural Partnership (SEMAP). SEMAP is dedicated to preserving and expanding access to local food and sustainable farming in Southeastern Massachusetts through research and education, Farmers Market Guide, https://semaponline.org/

Sierra Club, Iowa Chapter, Sustainable Agriculture Glossary, PDF, https://www.sierraclub.org

Sierra Club, Massachusetts Chapter, over 45-year legacy of protecting the environment with successful legislative, advocacy, and educational campaigns in Massachusetts, https://www.sierraclub.org/massachusetts/about

Sustainable Table, Sustainable Table celebrates local, sustainable food, educates consumers about the benefits of sustainable agriculture and works to build community through food, Grace Communications Foundation, food, food program, http://www.sustainabletable.org/

The Organic Food Guide, your source for organic and sustainable products across Massachusetts, Find Farms, https://www.theorganicfoodguide.org/

Time Health, Health Diet/Nutrition, http://time.com/

University of California Cooperative Extension, Horticulture and Small Farms, Glossary of Terms, http://ucanr.edu/sites/ceplacerhorticulture/EatLocal/Glossary/

United States Department of Agriculture, USDA, Agriculture Marketing Services, and National Agricultural Statistics Service, data and statistics, https://www.ams.usda.gov

United States Food and Drug Administration, US FDA, the US Department of Health and Human Services, https://www.fda.gov/

Visit New England, Visit Massachusetts, Massachusetts, State, food & Drink, Farmers Markets, Massachusetts farmers markets sell local food, authentic crafts, http://www.visit-massachusetts.com/state/farmers-market

[i] USDA, United States Department of Agriculture, Agricultural Marketing Service, Organic Labeling, Organic Regulations, Home>Rules & regulations, https://www.ams.usda.gov/rules-regulations/organic/labeling

[ii] Silverbrook Farm, website, info, sustainable farming, http://www.silverbrookdartmouth.com/new-page/

[iii] Certified Naturally Grown, Declaration for 2018, "For Farmers", https://certified.naturallygrown.org/documents/Declaration.pdf

[iv] Certified Naturally Grown, Allowed & Prohibited Substances, https://www.cngfarming.org/alprosubstances

[v] Consumer Reports, Greener Choices, Labels, Food Labels, We Evaluate and rate food labels so you can make informed decisions, http://greenerchoices.org/labels/

[vi] Food and Drug Administration, the US Department of Health and Human Services, website, https://www.fda.gov/Food/IngredientsPackagingLabeling/GEPlants/ucm461805.ht m

[vii] Food and Drug Administration, the US Department of Health and Human Services, website, https://www.fda.gov/Food/IngredientsPackagingLabeling/GEPlants/ucm461805.ht m

[viii] Time, Health Diet/Nutrition, These charts show every genetically modified food people already eat in the U.S., by David JOHNSON and SIOBHAN O'CONNOR April 30, 2015; http://time.com/3840073/gmo-food-charts/

[ix] GMO Answers, GMO Answers was created to do a better job answering your questions — no matter what they are — about GMOs. Current GMO crops, https://gmoanswers.com/current-gmo-crops

[x] Living non-gmo, a lifestyle site created by the non-gmo project, https://livingnongmo.org/learn/resources/

[xi] Florida Department of Agriculture and Consumer Services, Divisions & Offices, Marketing and development, Consumer Resources, Buy "Fresh from Florida", Crops in Season, https://www.freshfromflorida.com/Divisions-Offices/Marketing-and-Development/Consumer-Resources/Buy-Fresh-From-Florida/Crops-in-Season

[xii] One Green Planet, Welcome to Green Monsters! We're your online guide to making conscious choices that help people, animals and the planet, How to choose a papaya that's not genetically modified, Heather McClees, June 19, 2017, http://www.onegreenplanet.org/vegan-food/how-to-choose-a-papaya-thats-not-genetically-modified/

[xiii] USDA, United States Department of Agriculture, National Agricultural Statistics Service, data and statistics, https://www.nass.usda.gov/Charts_and_Maps/Crops_County/sb-pr.php

[xiv] SEMAP, Southeastern Massachusetts Agricultural Partnership, Southeastern MA harvest Calendar, Find the freshest locally grown fruits, vegetables, dairy, and meats at your local farmers market or farmstand, southeastern ma vegetables, https://guide.farmfreshri.org/learn/harvestcalendar.php,

[xv] Grace Communications Foundation Inc., Seasonal Food Guide, Find what's in season near you, Massachusetts Seasonal Food Guide, https://www.seasonalfoodguide.org/massachusetts/

[xvi] Massachusetts Department of Agricultural Resources, Massachusetts-Grown Produce availability Calendar, http://www.stoughtonfarmersmarket.org/uploads/5/8/6/4/58641259/availability-chart.pdf